The BOOGER BOOK

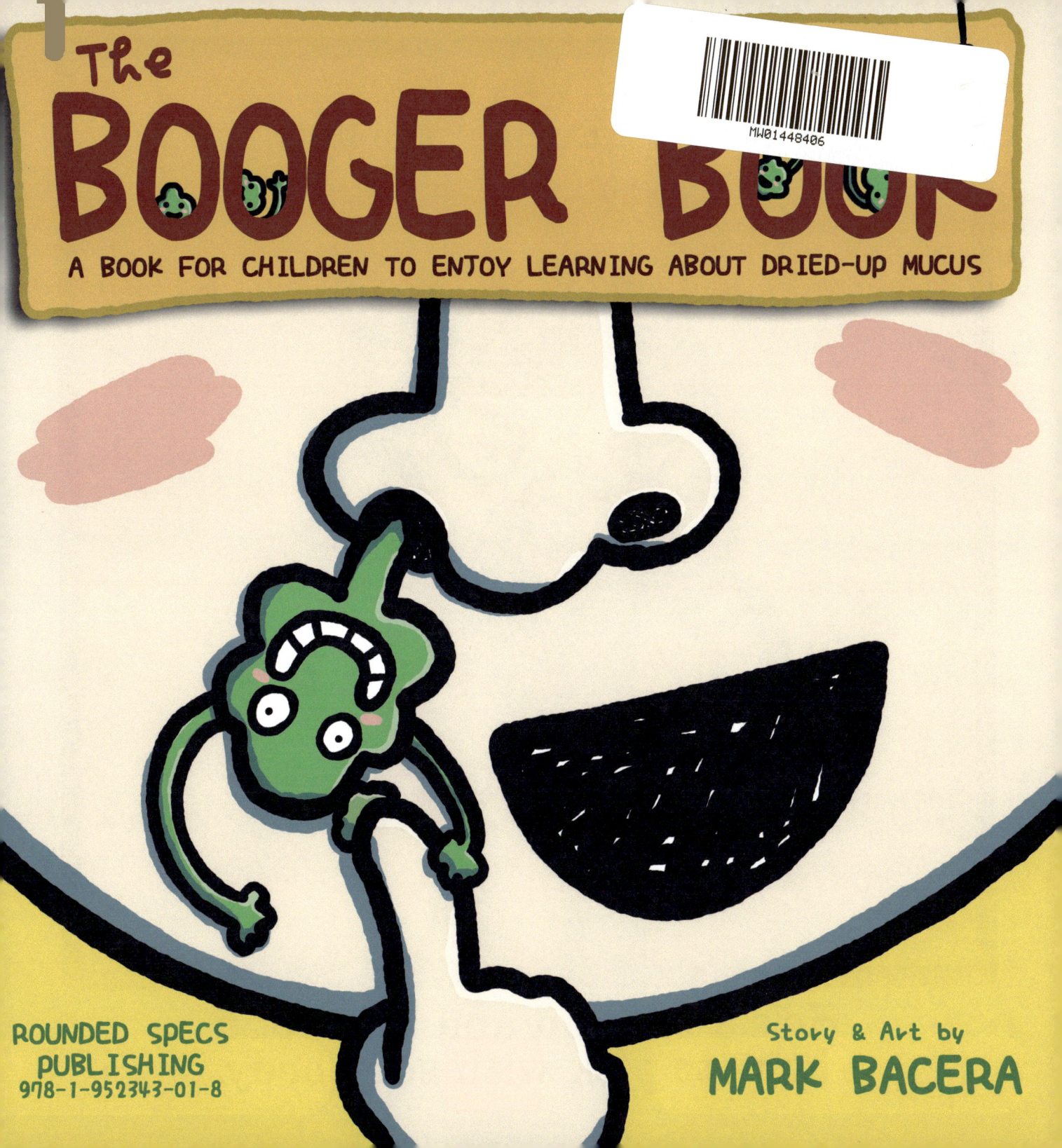

A BOOK FOR CHILDREN TO ENJOY LEARNING ABOUT DRIED-UP MUCUS

ROUNDED SPECS
PUBLISHING
978-1-952343-01-8

Story & Art by
MARK BACERA

Look! It's Bueller, the bully.

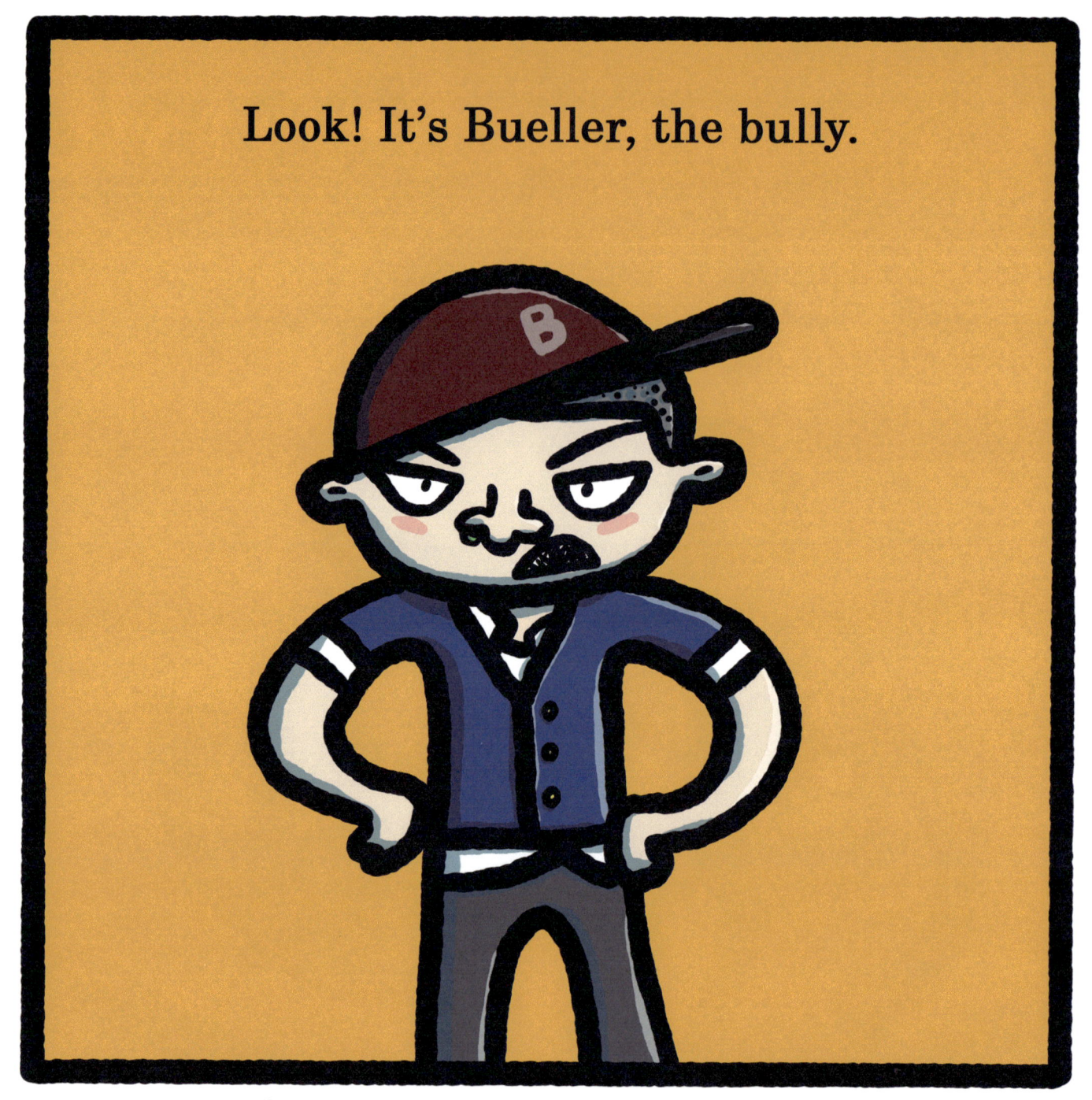

He's a bad kid and he's got a bone to pick with somebody.

Oh wait...
No...

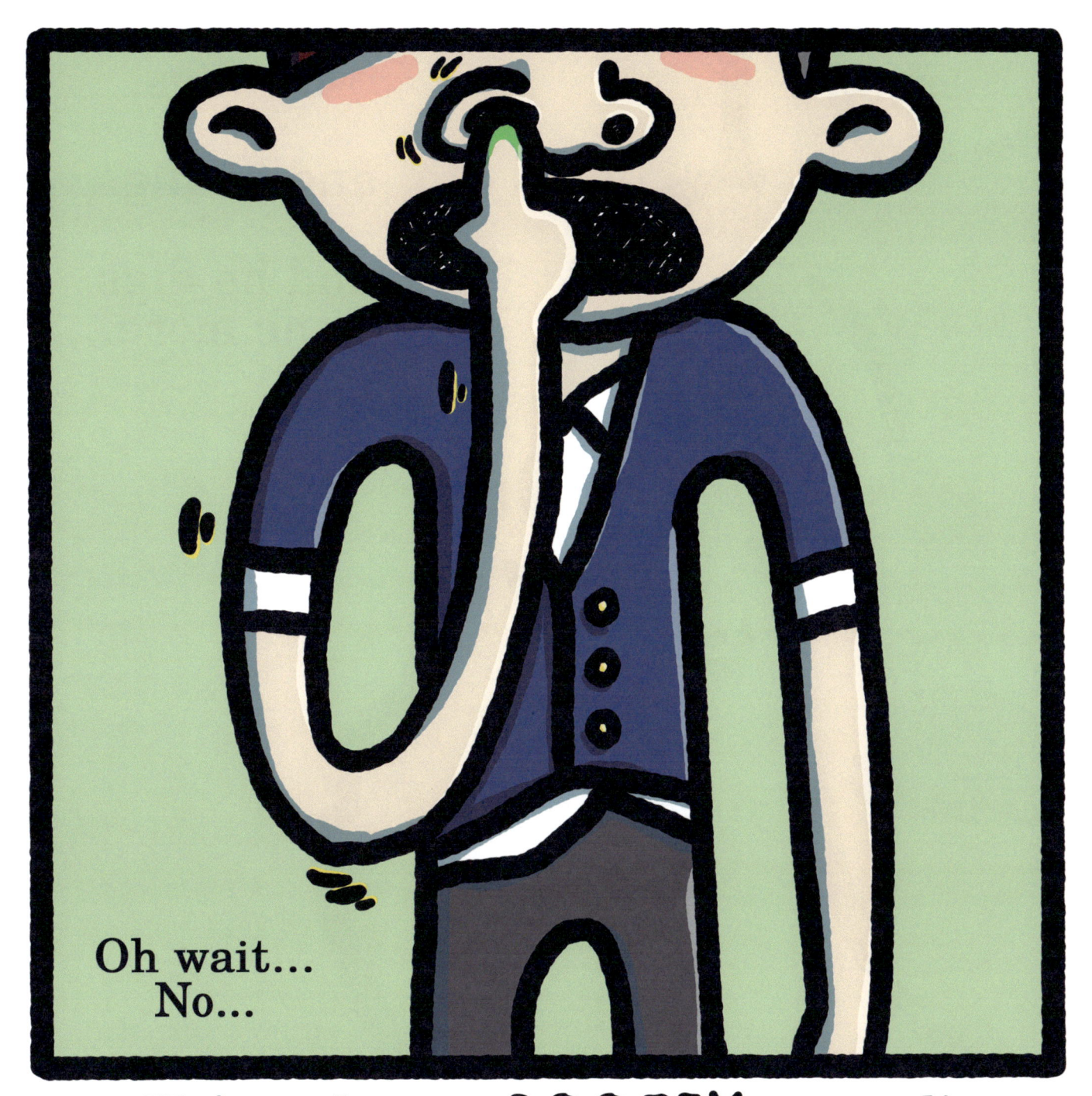

He's picking a **BOOGEY** instead!
Here he goes...

He digs,

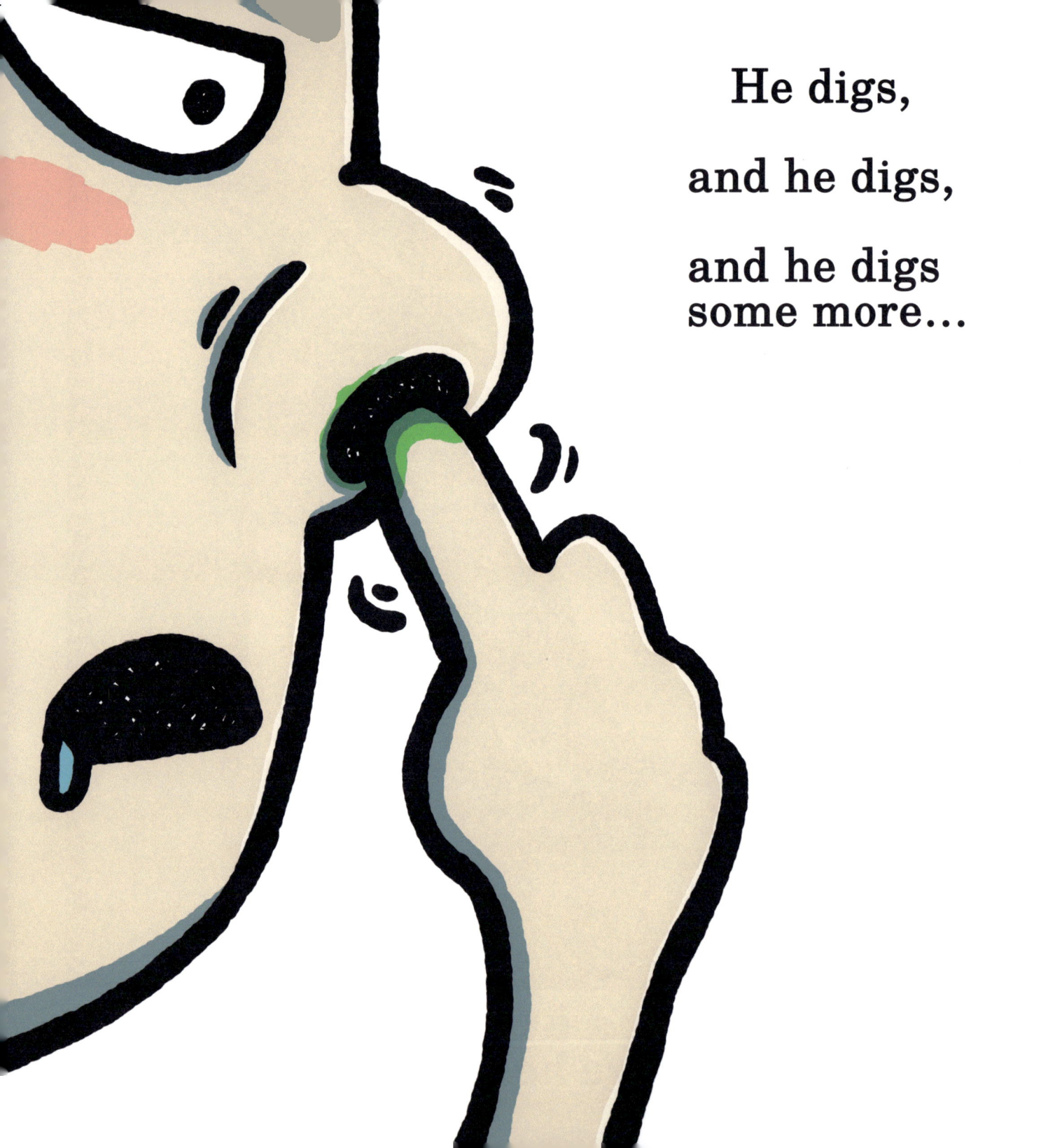

and he digs,

and he digs some more...

Ah—
He's found something!

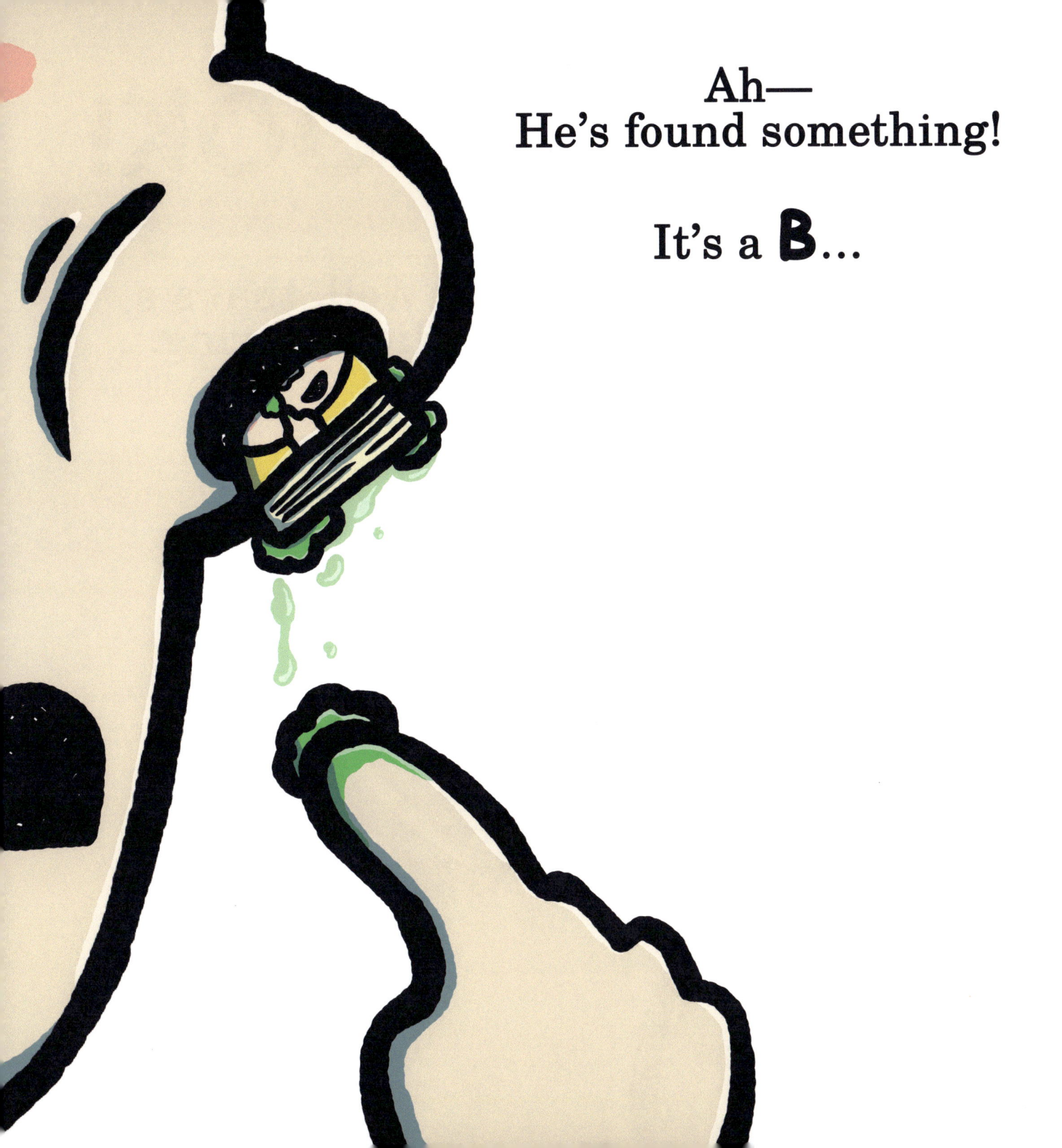

It's a **B**...

BOOK!

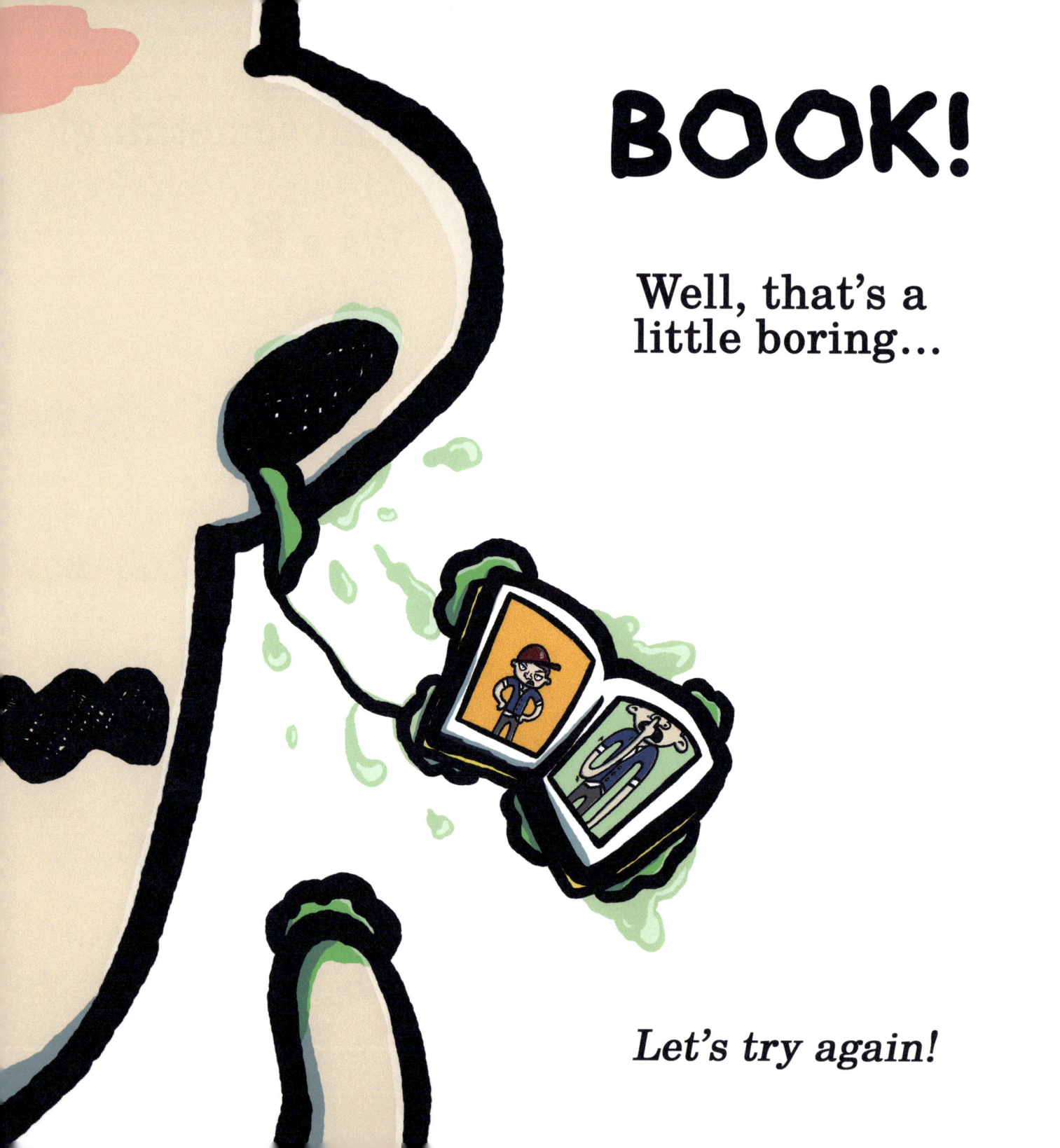

Well, that's a little boring...

Let's try again!

Ah—
He's found something!

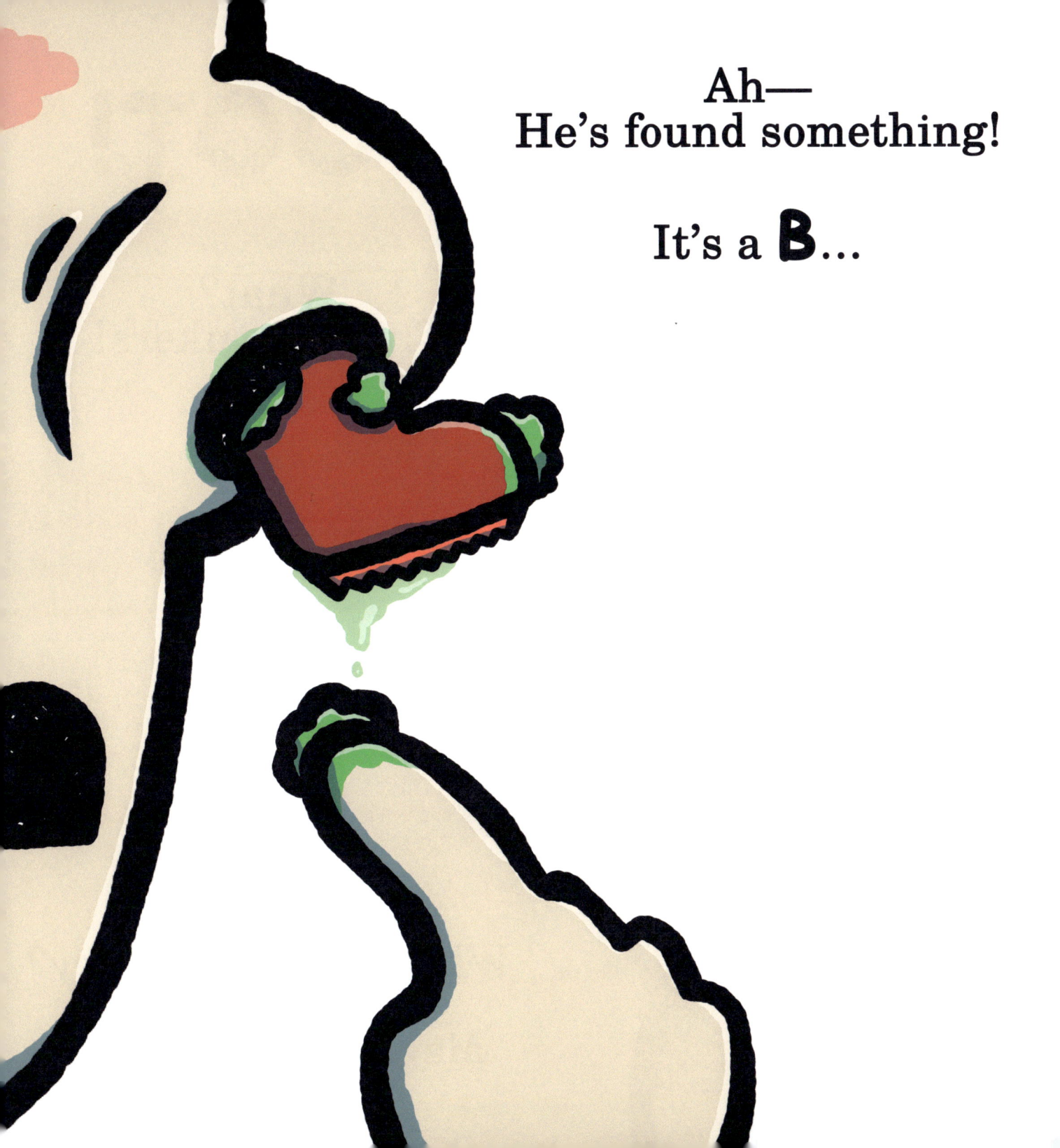

It's a **B**...

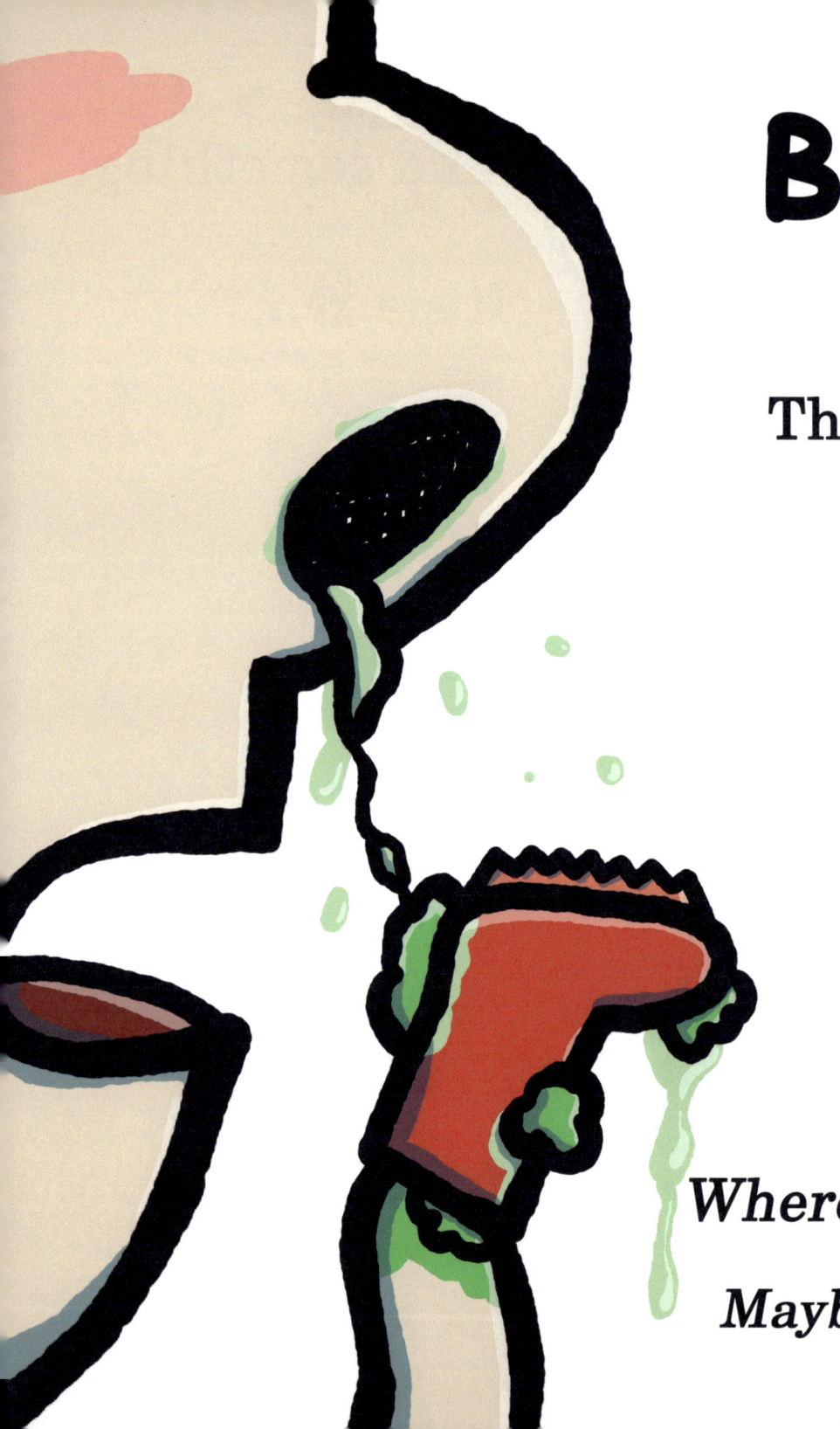

BOOT!

What?
This is bonkers!

Where is that boogey?

Maybe the next one...

Ah—
He's found something!

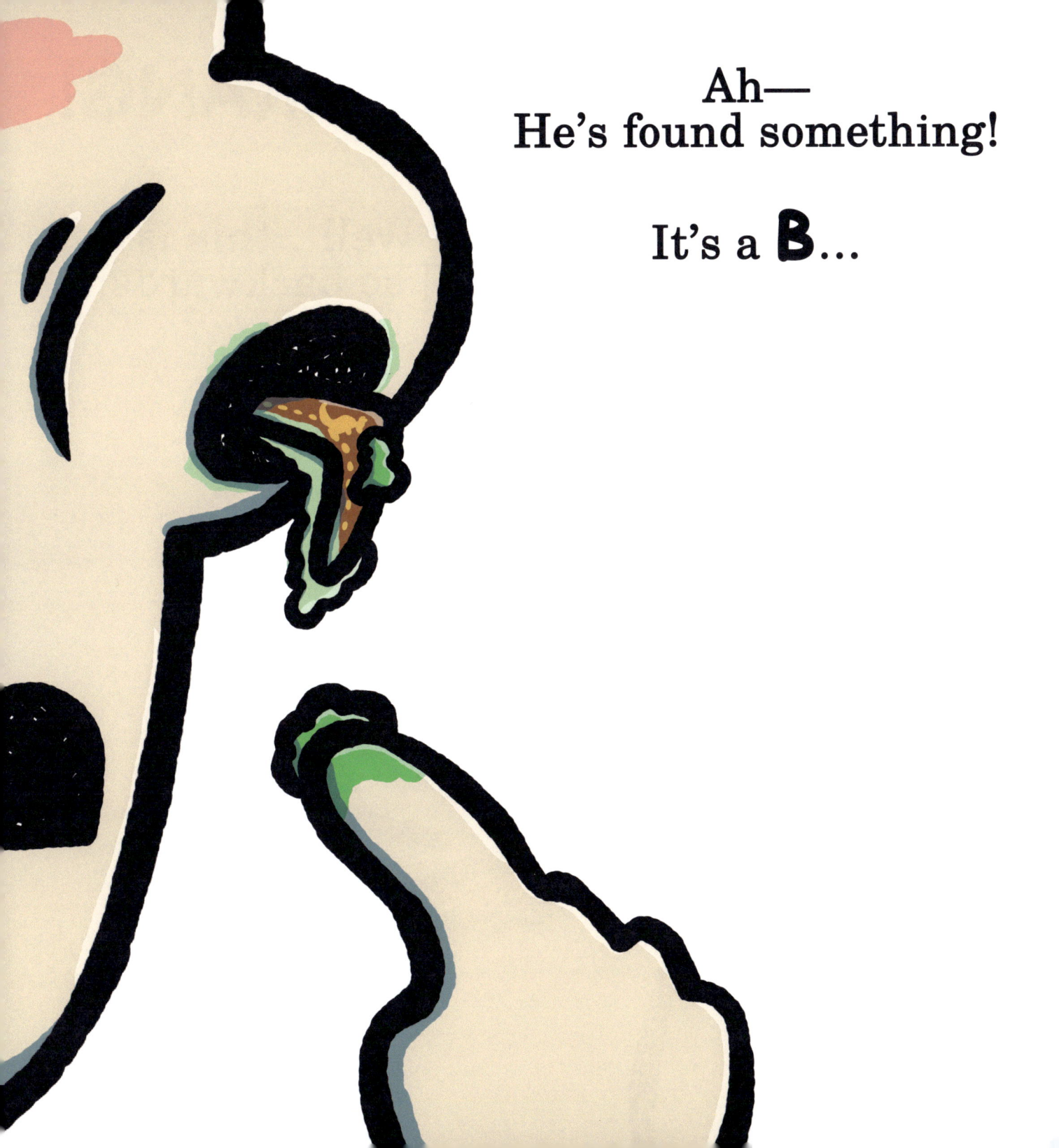

It's a **B**...

BOOMERANG!

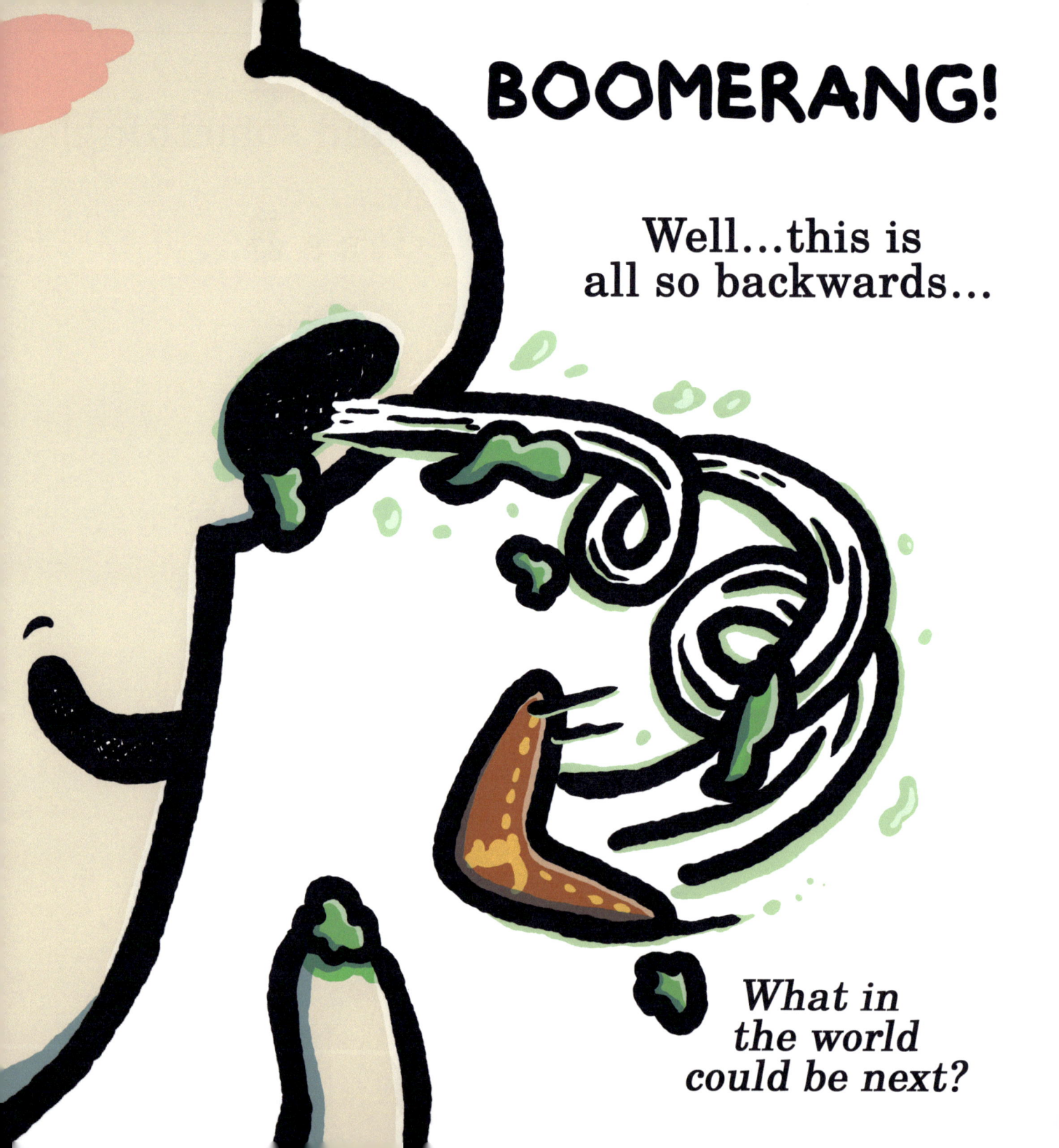

Well...this is all so backwards...

What in the world could be next?

Ah—
He's found something!

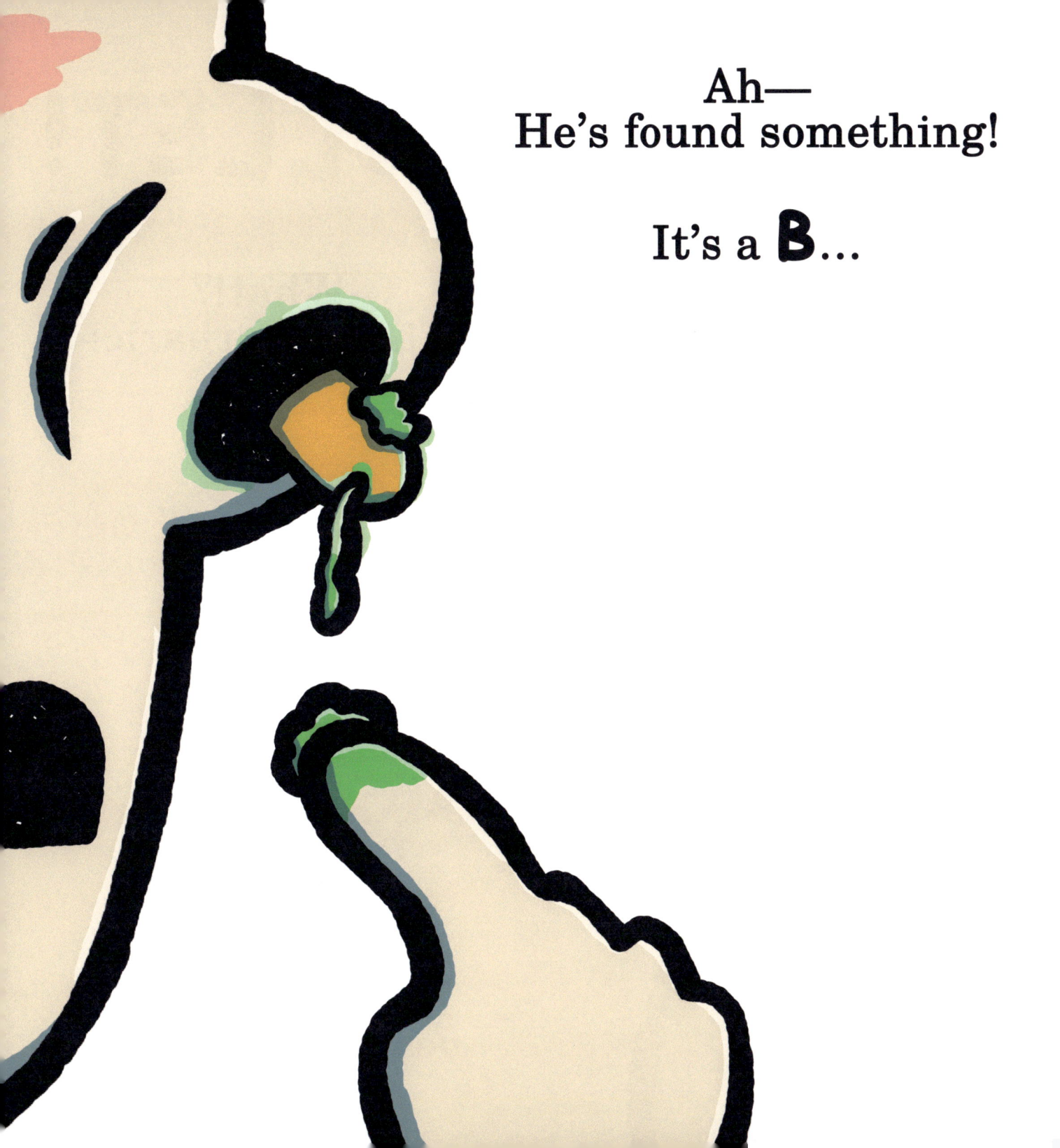

It's a **B**...

BULLET!

What!?
This is barbaric!

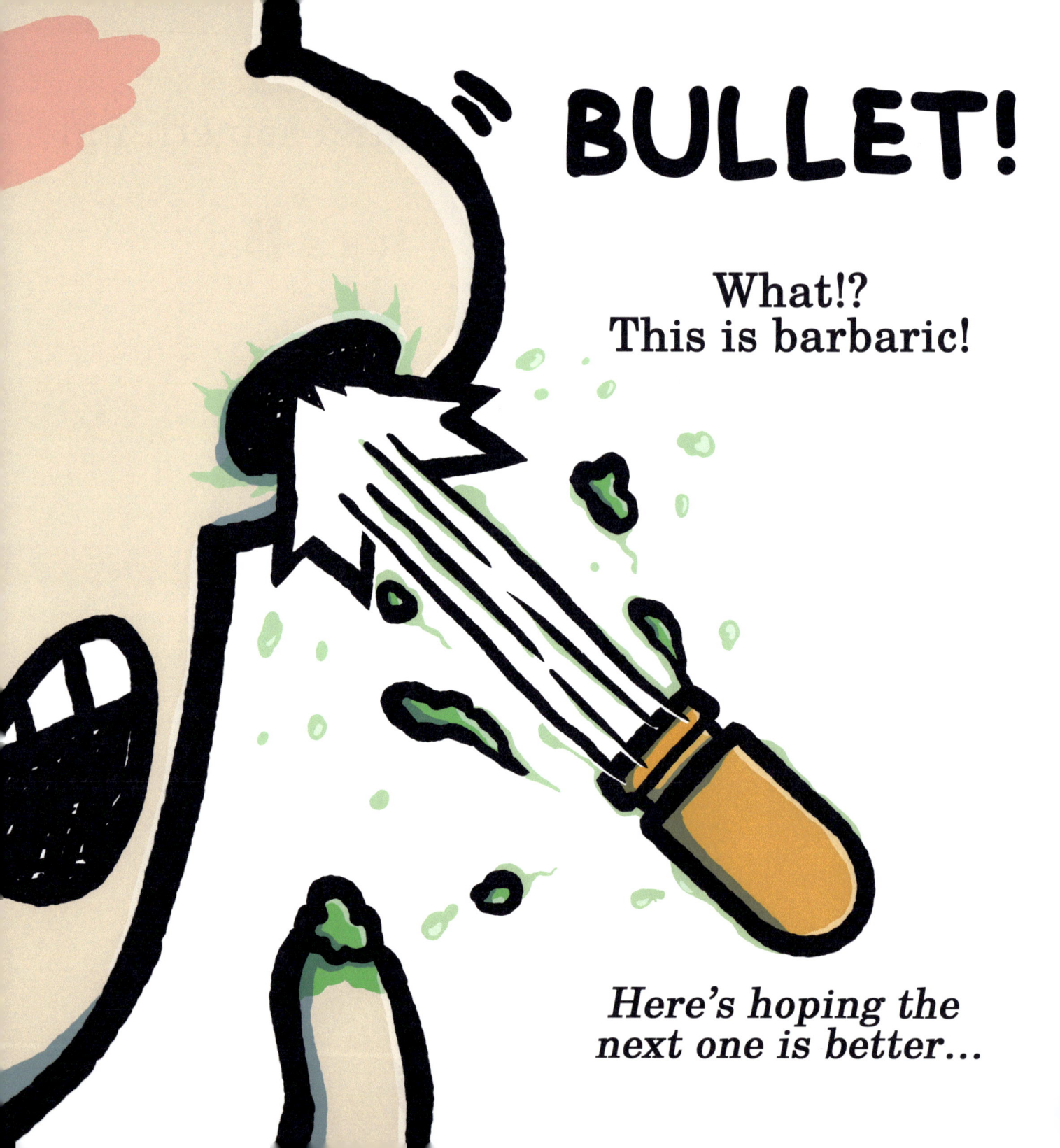

Here's hoping the
next one is better...

Ah—
He's found something!

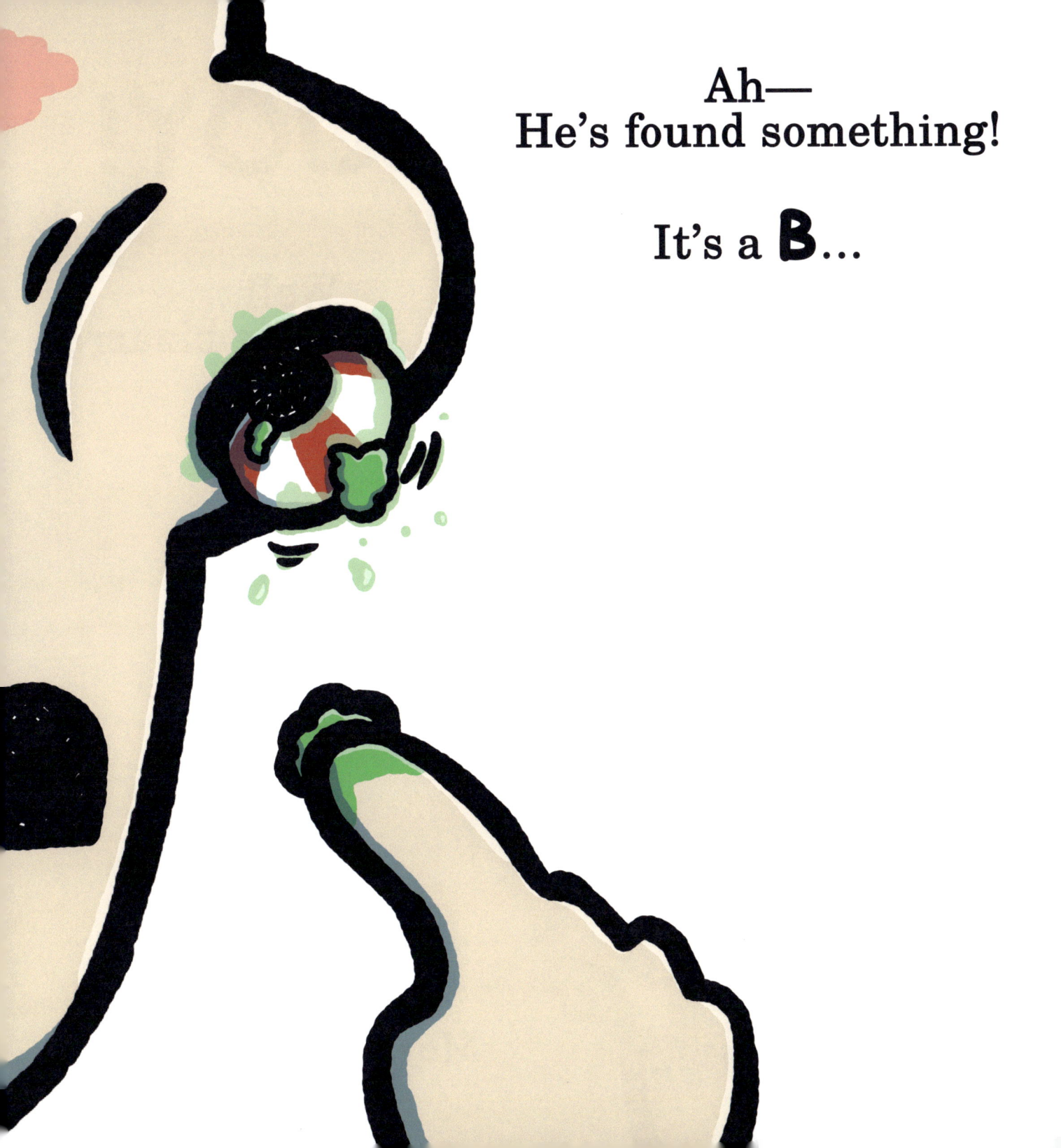

It's a **B**…

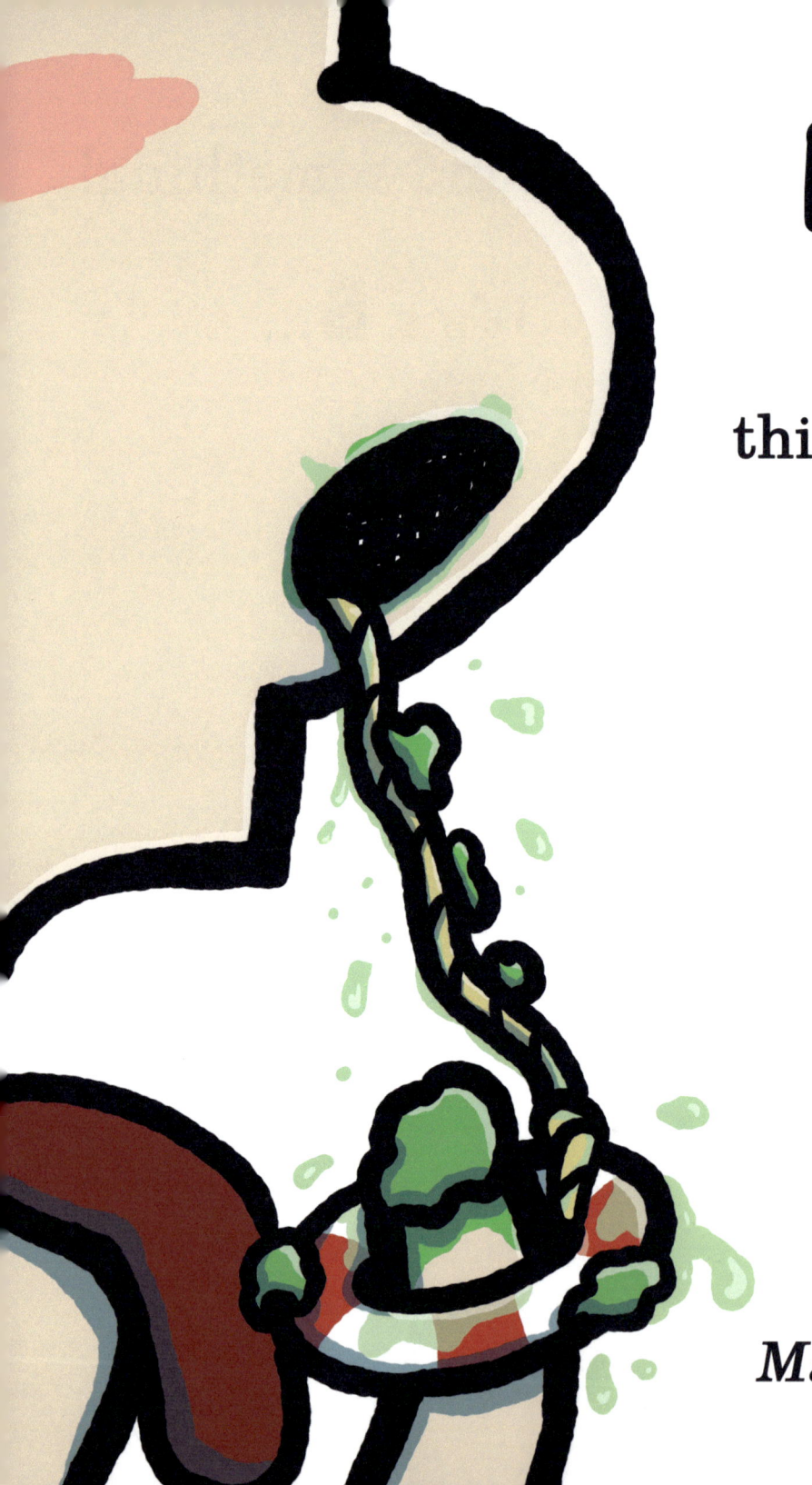

BUOY!

Well...
this is quite bizarre.

Maybe, just maybe...

Ah—
He's found something!

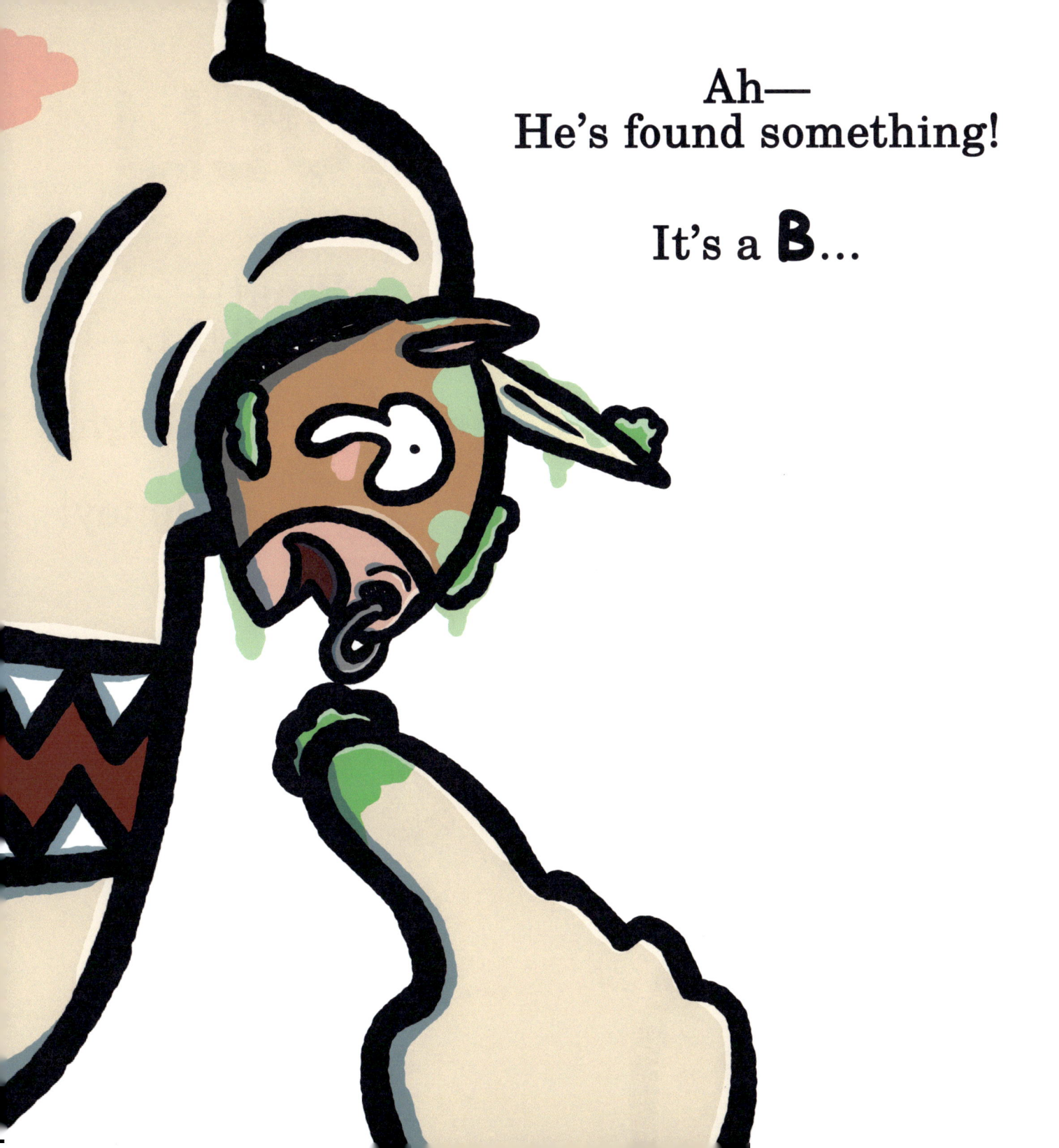

It's a **B**...

BULL!

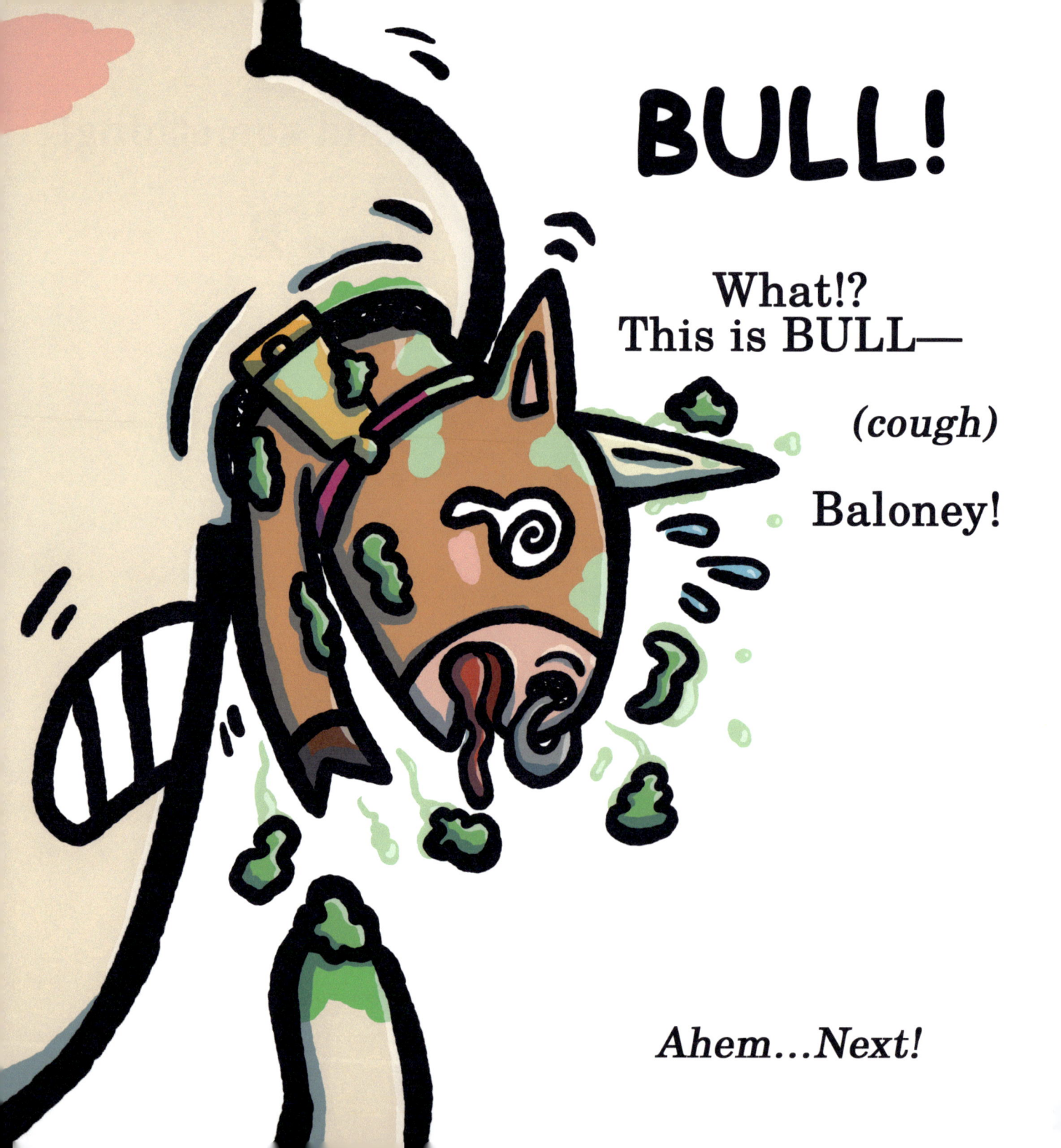

What!?
This is BULL—

(cough)

Baloney!

Ahem...Next!

Ah—
He's found something!

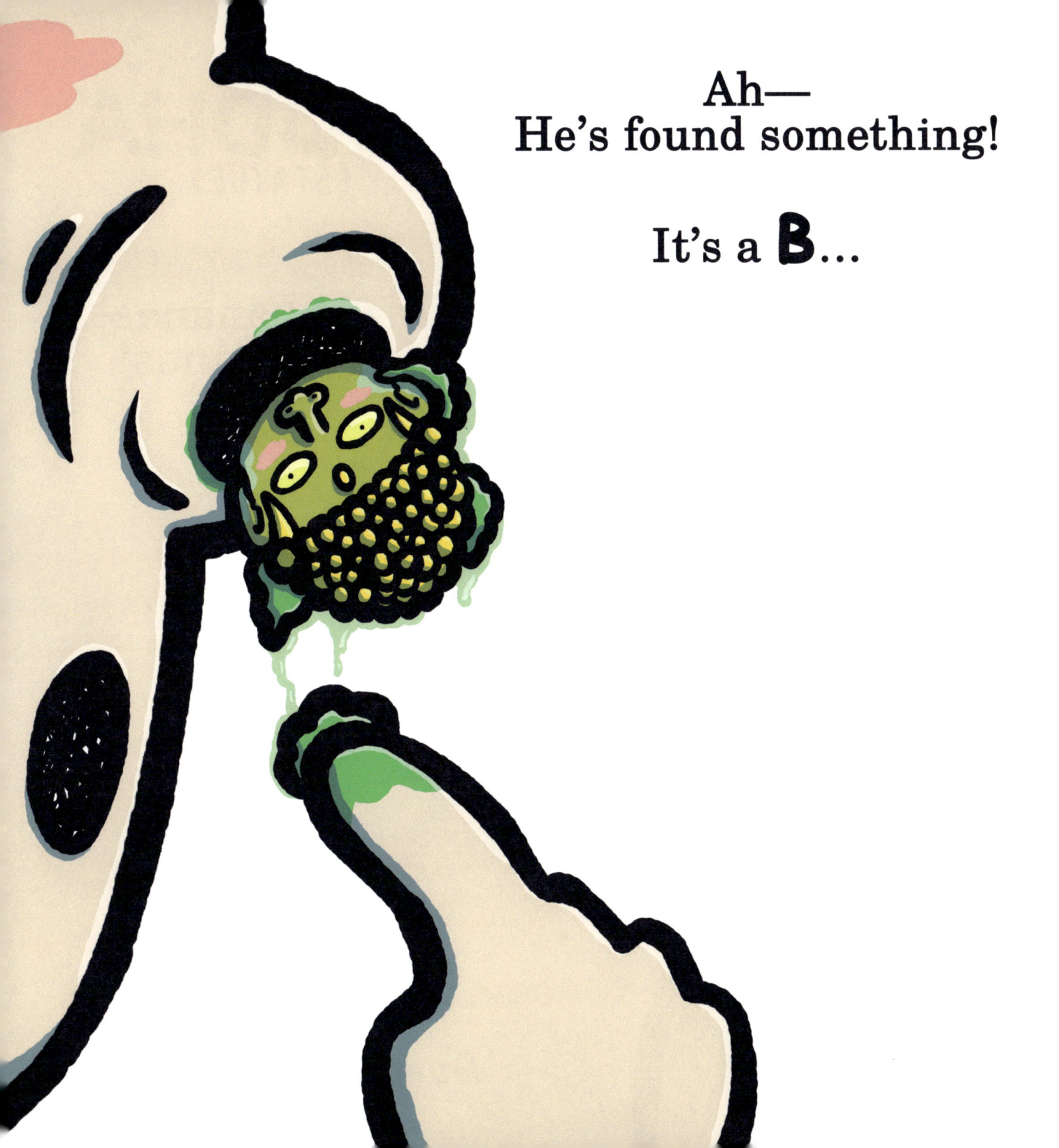

It's a **B**...

BUDDHA
(STATUE)

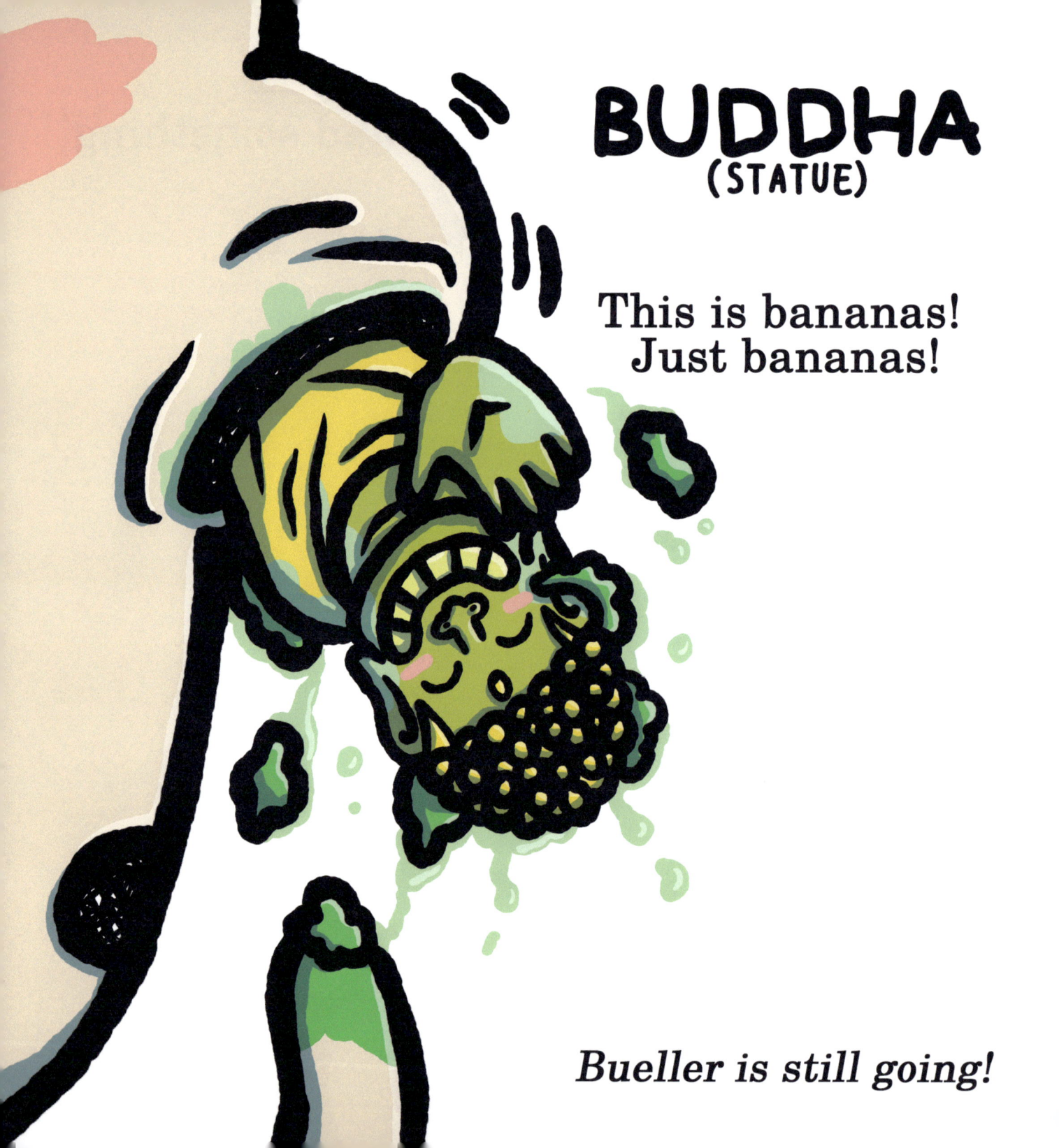

This is bananas!
Just bananas!

Bueller is still going!

Ah—
He's found something!

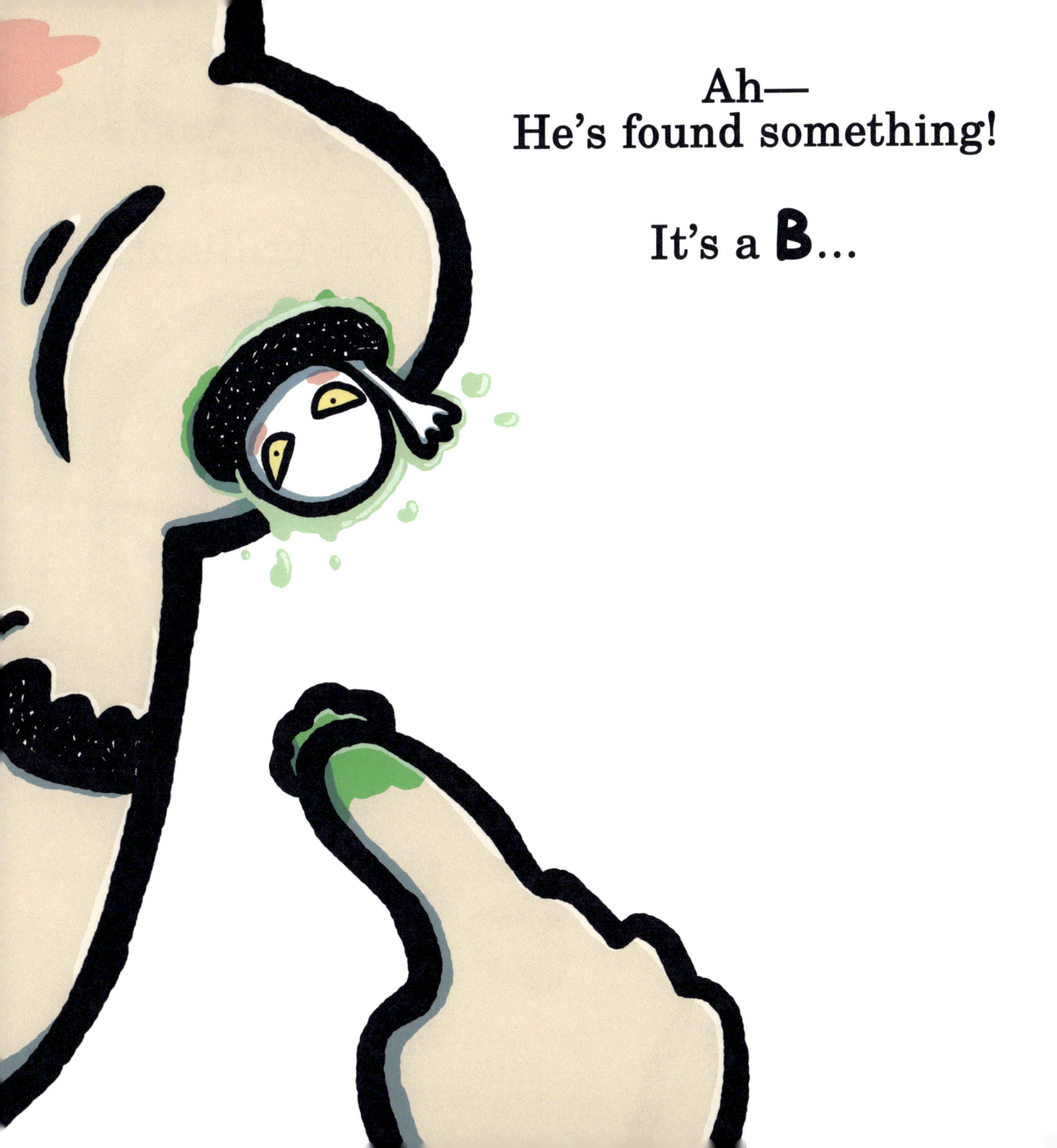

It's a **B**...

BOO!
(GHOST)

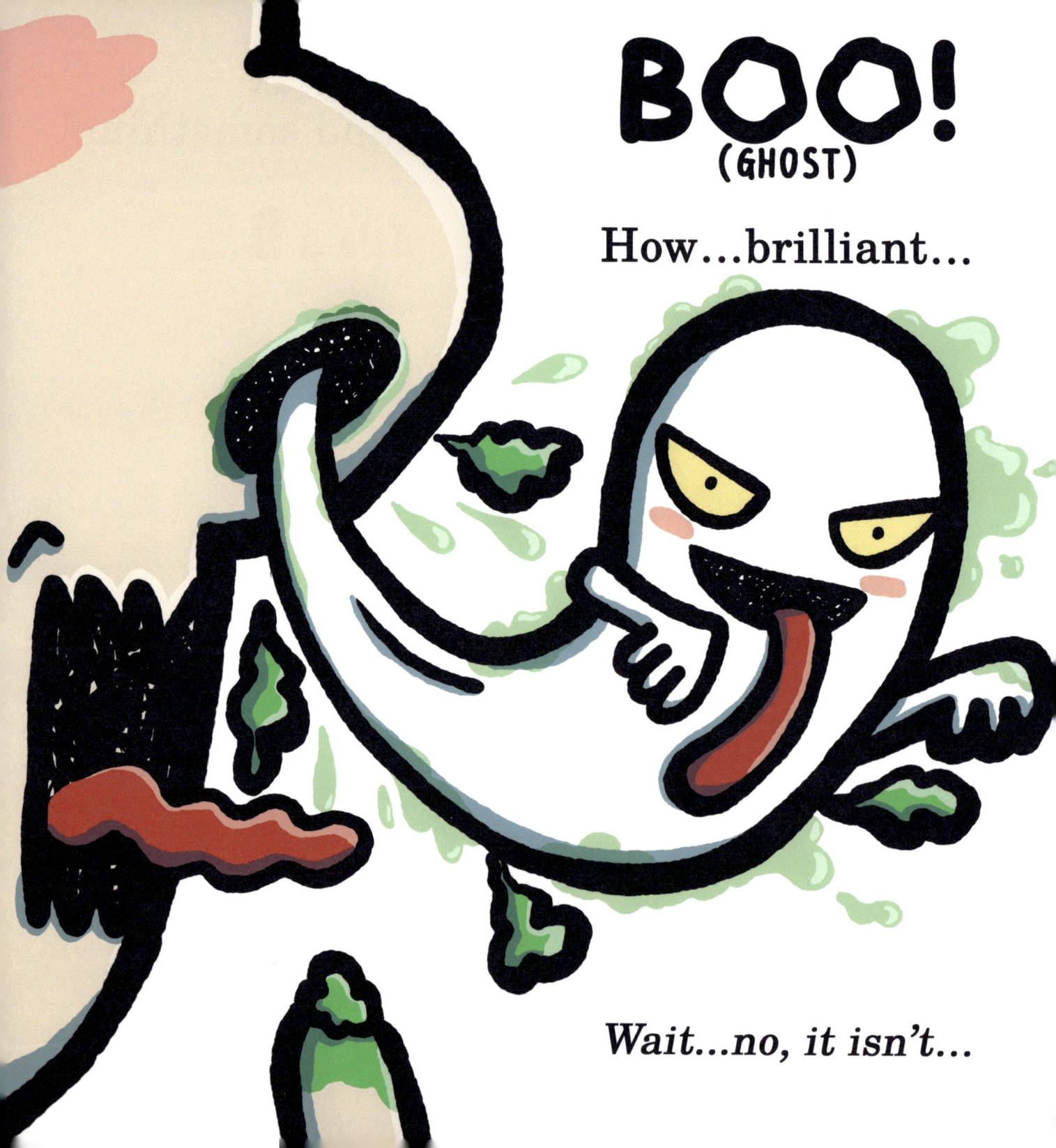

How...brilliant...

Wait...no, it isn't...

Ah—
He's found something!

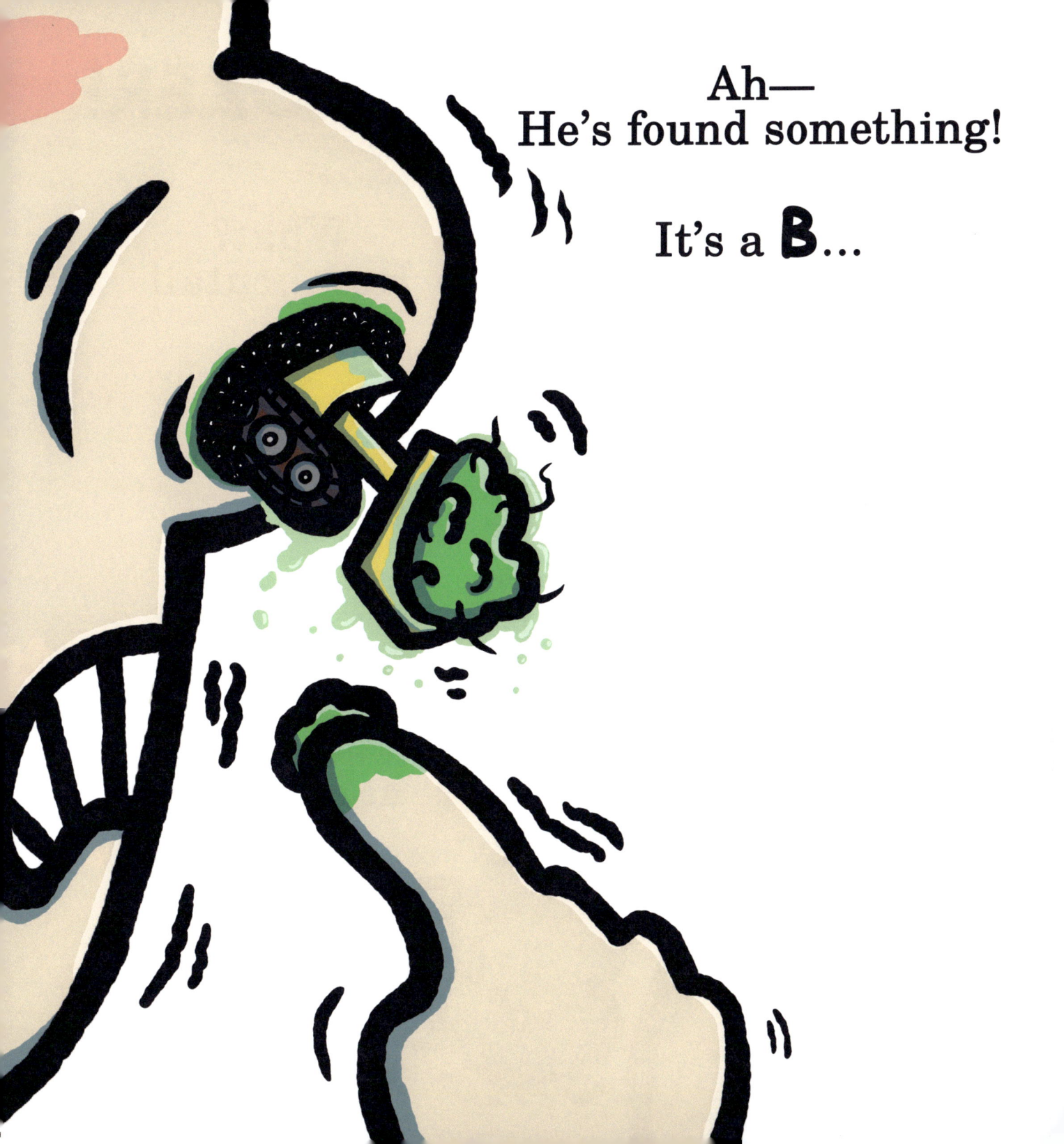

It's a **B**...

BULLDOZER!

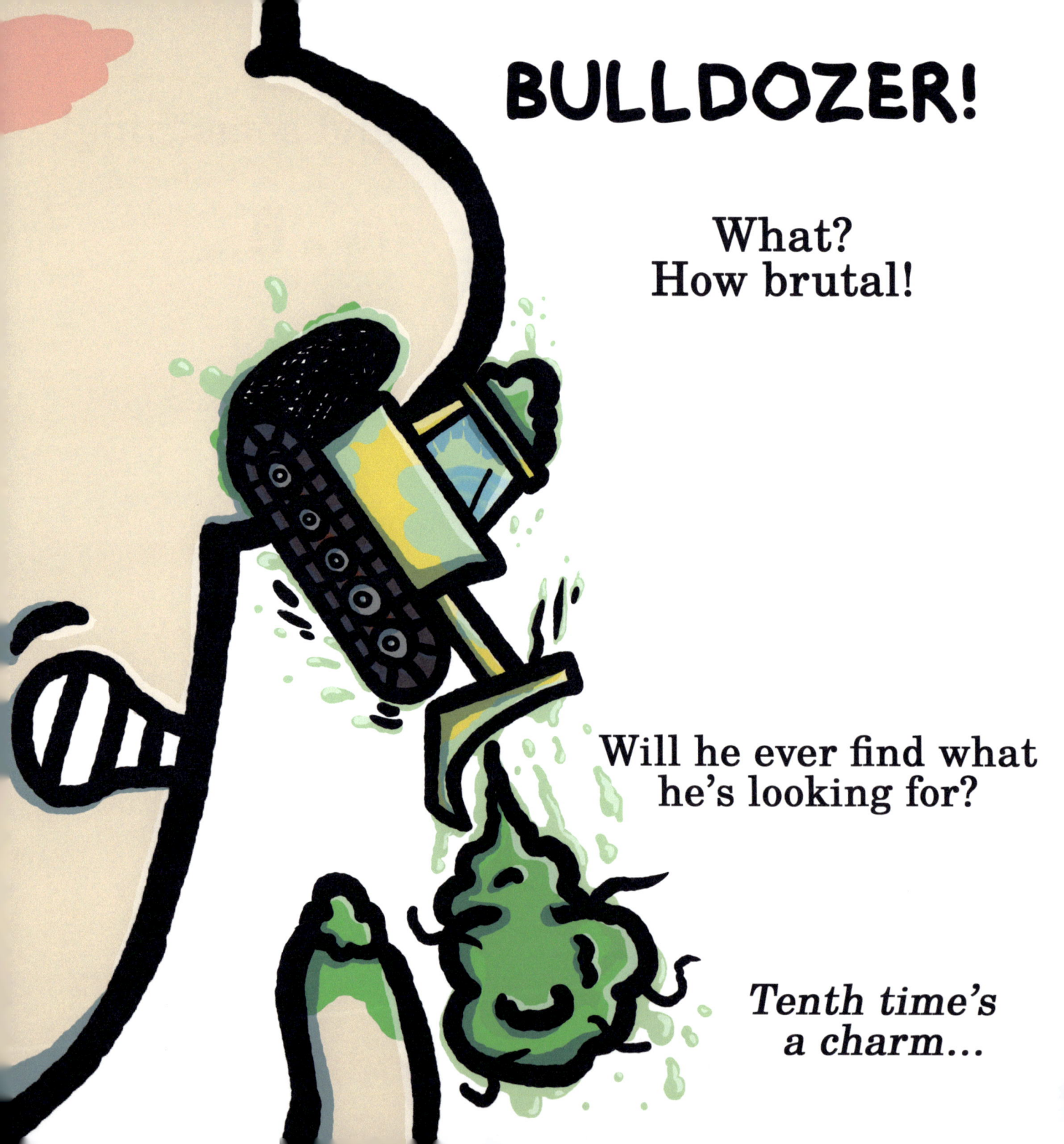

What?
How brutal!

Will he ever find what he's looking for?

Tenth time's a charm...

Ah—
He's found something!

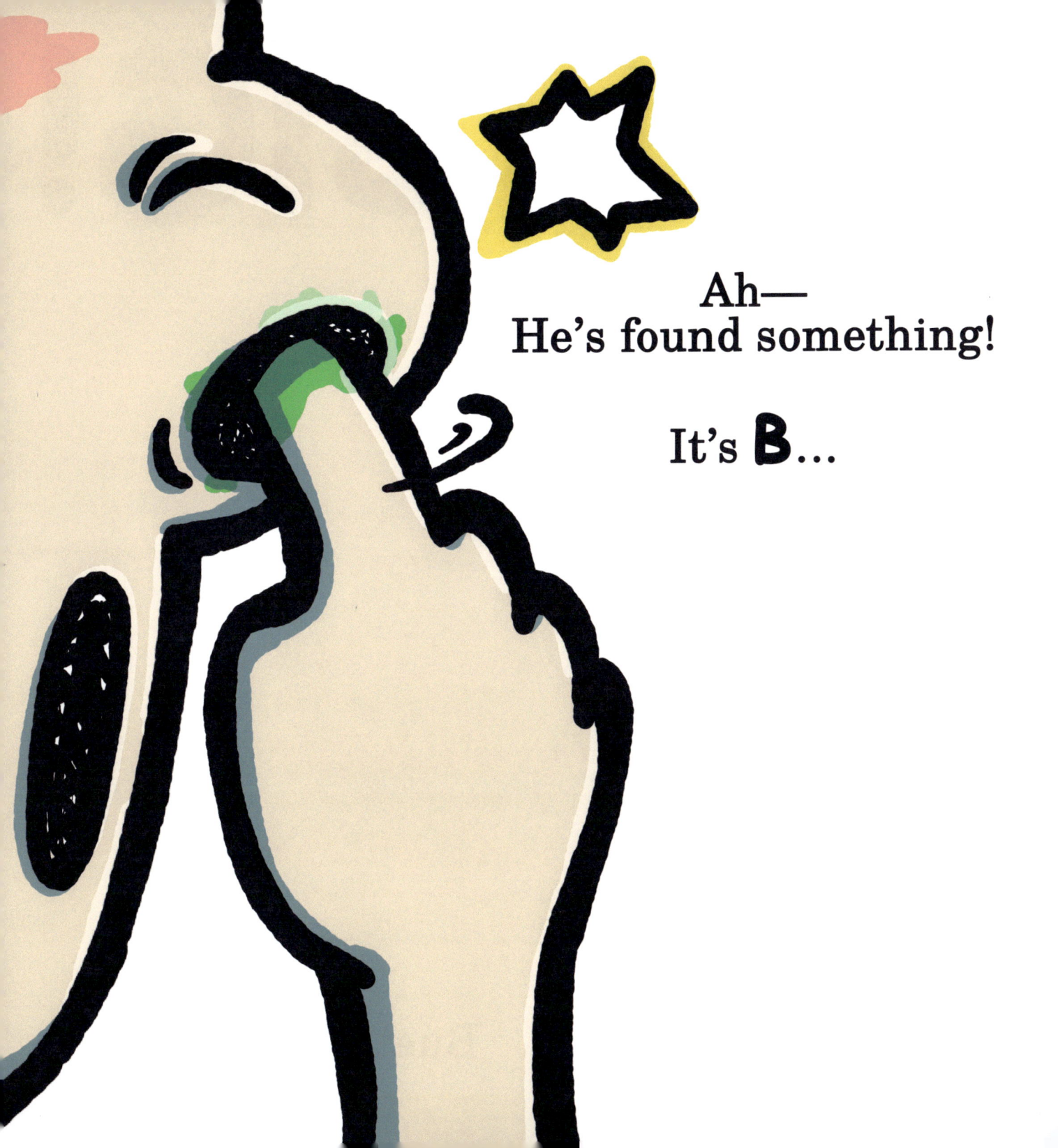

It's **B**...

BIG!

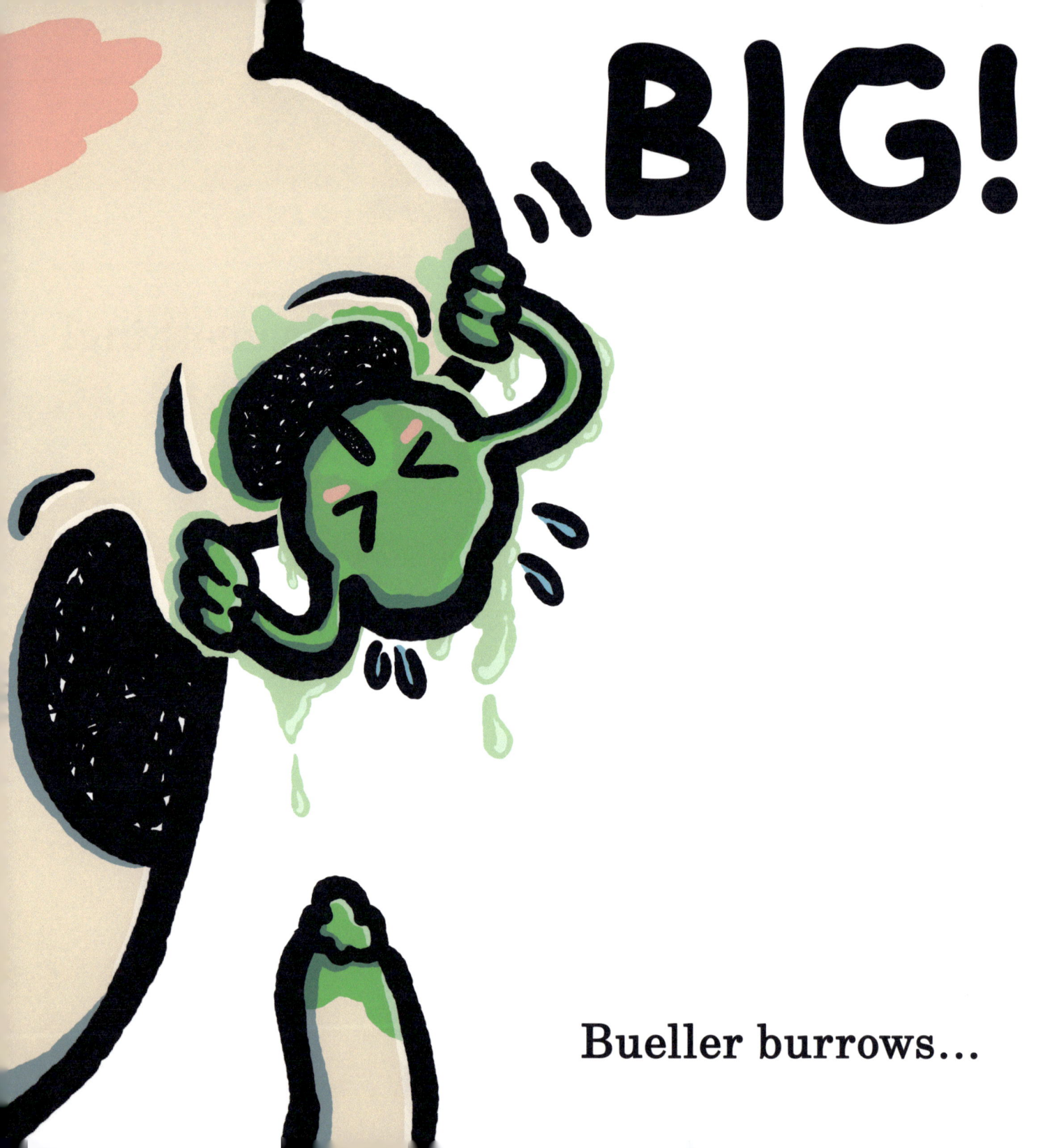

Bueller burrows...

...and he burrows...

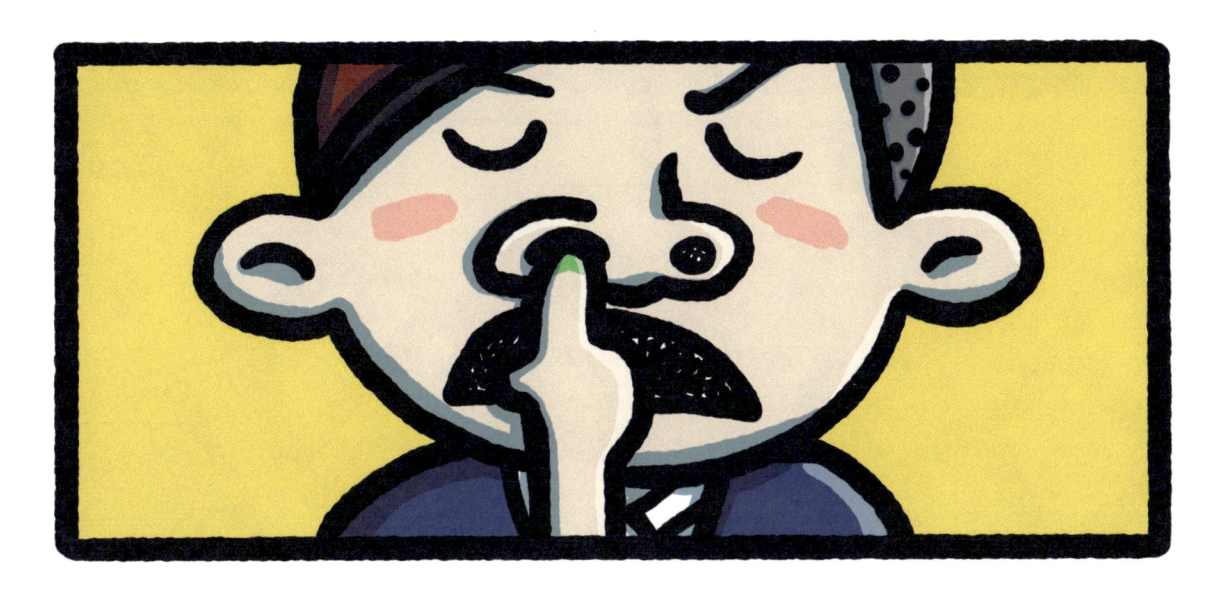

...and he burrows some more...

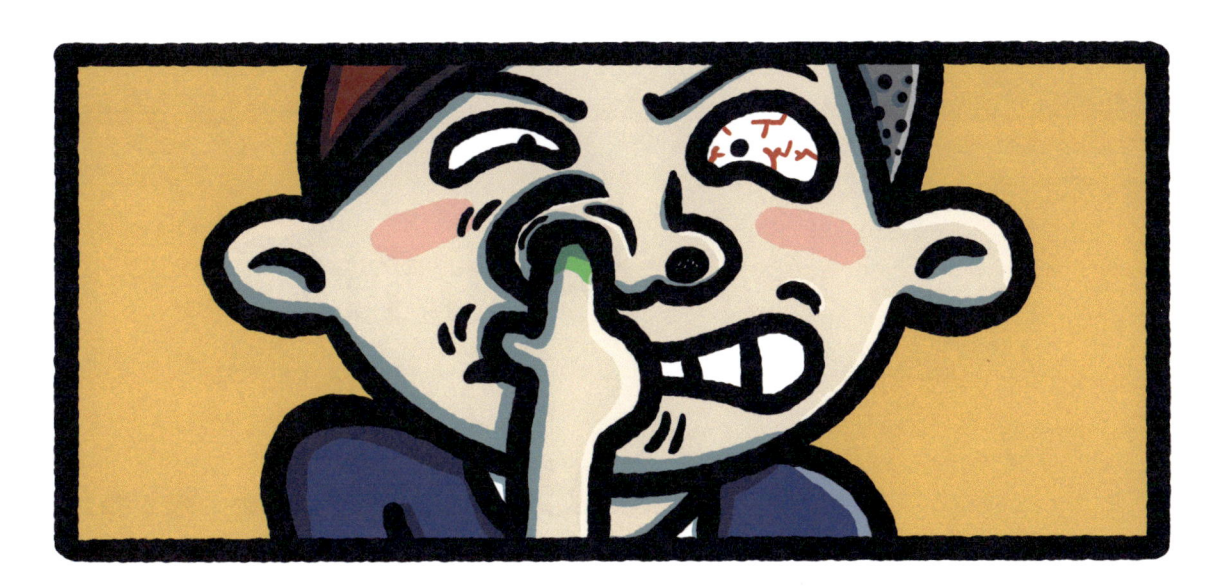

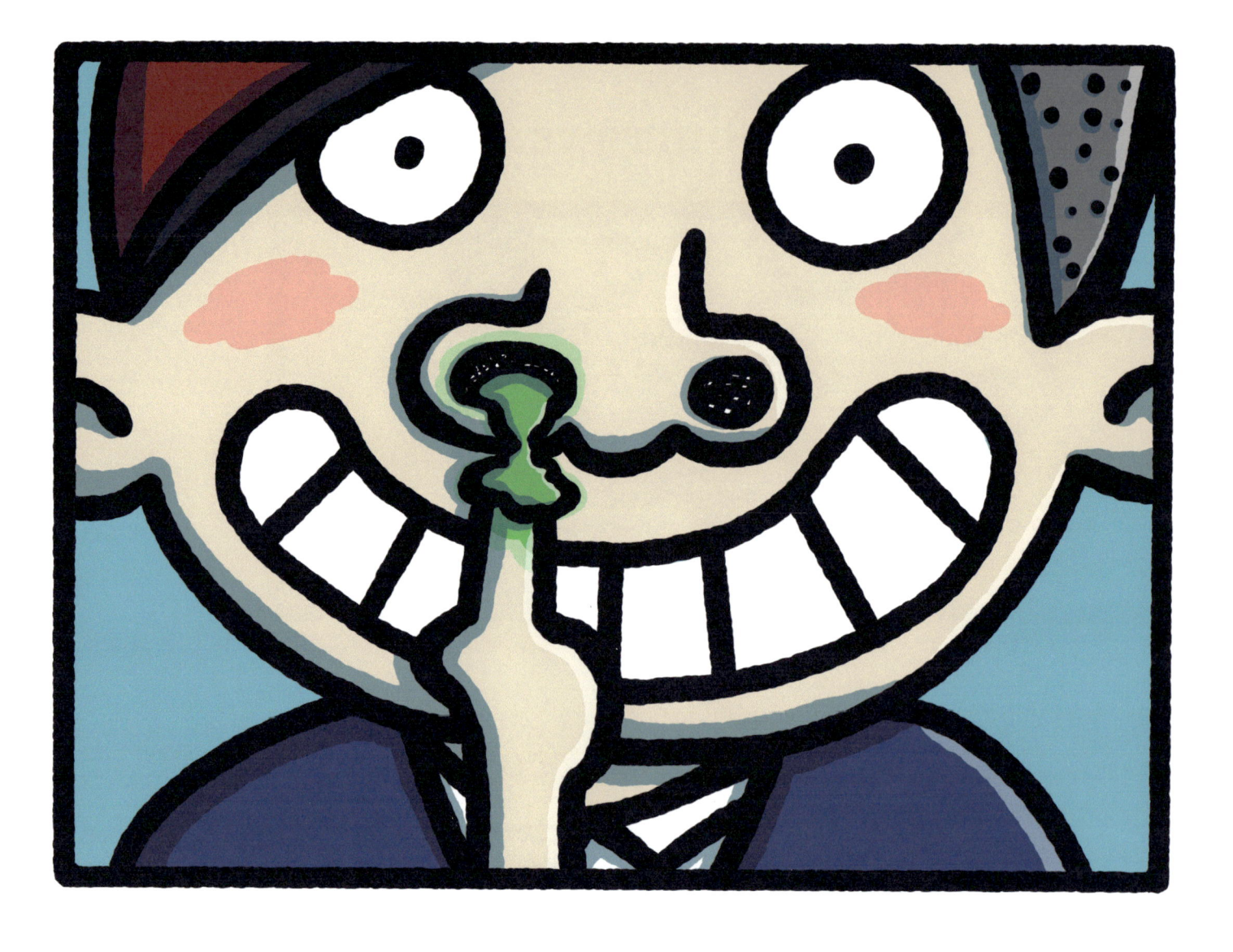

Got it!
It's a **B**...

FREE AT LAST!

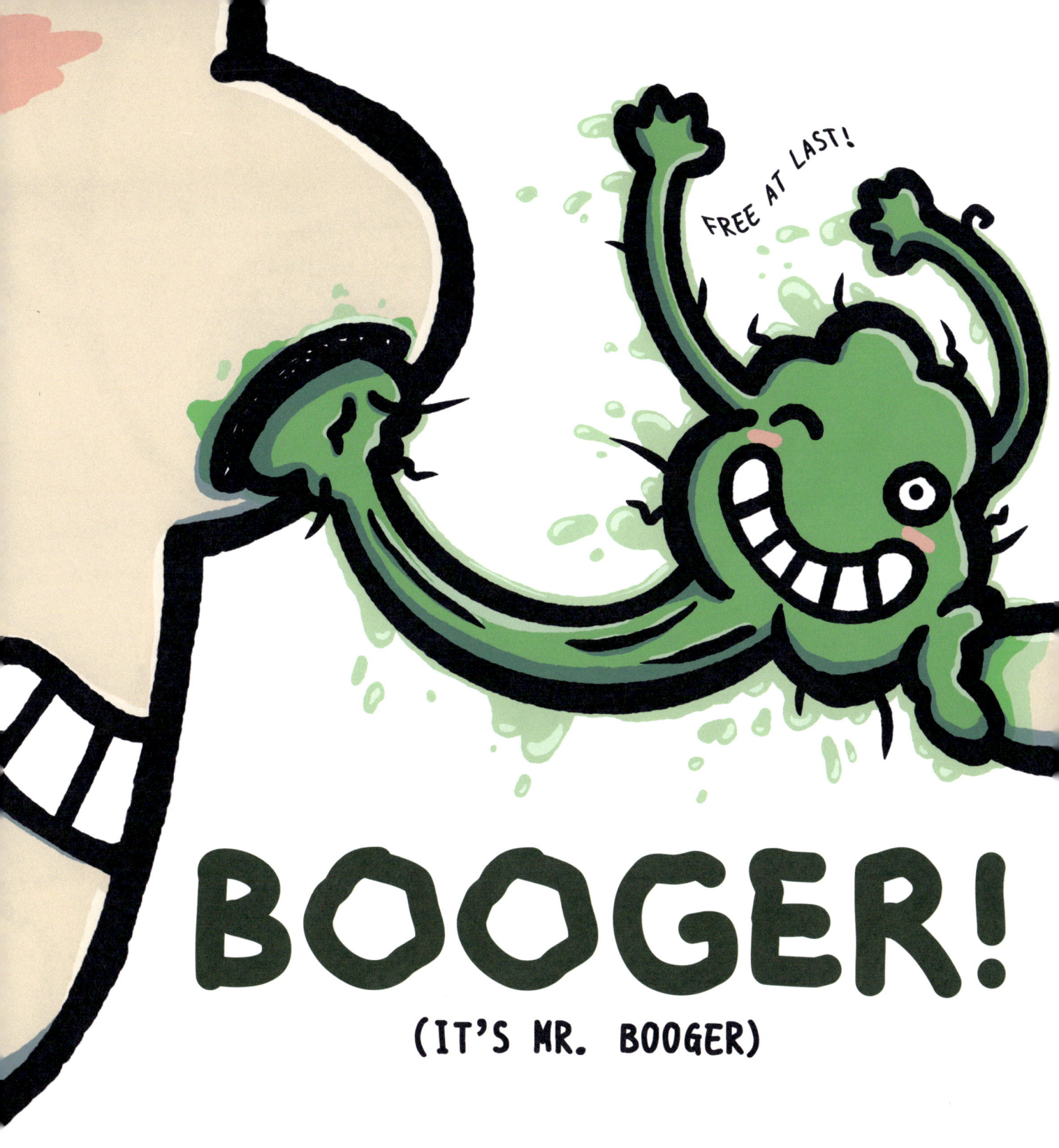

BOOGER!
(IT'S MR. BOOGER)

Ah—!
Don't eat him!

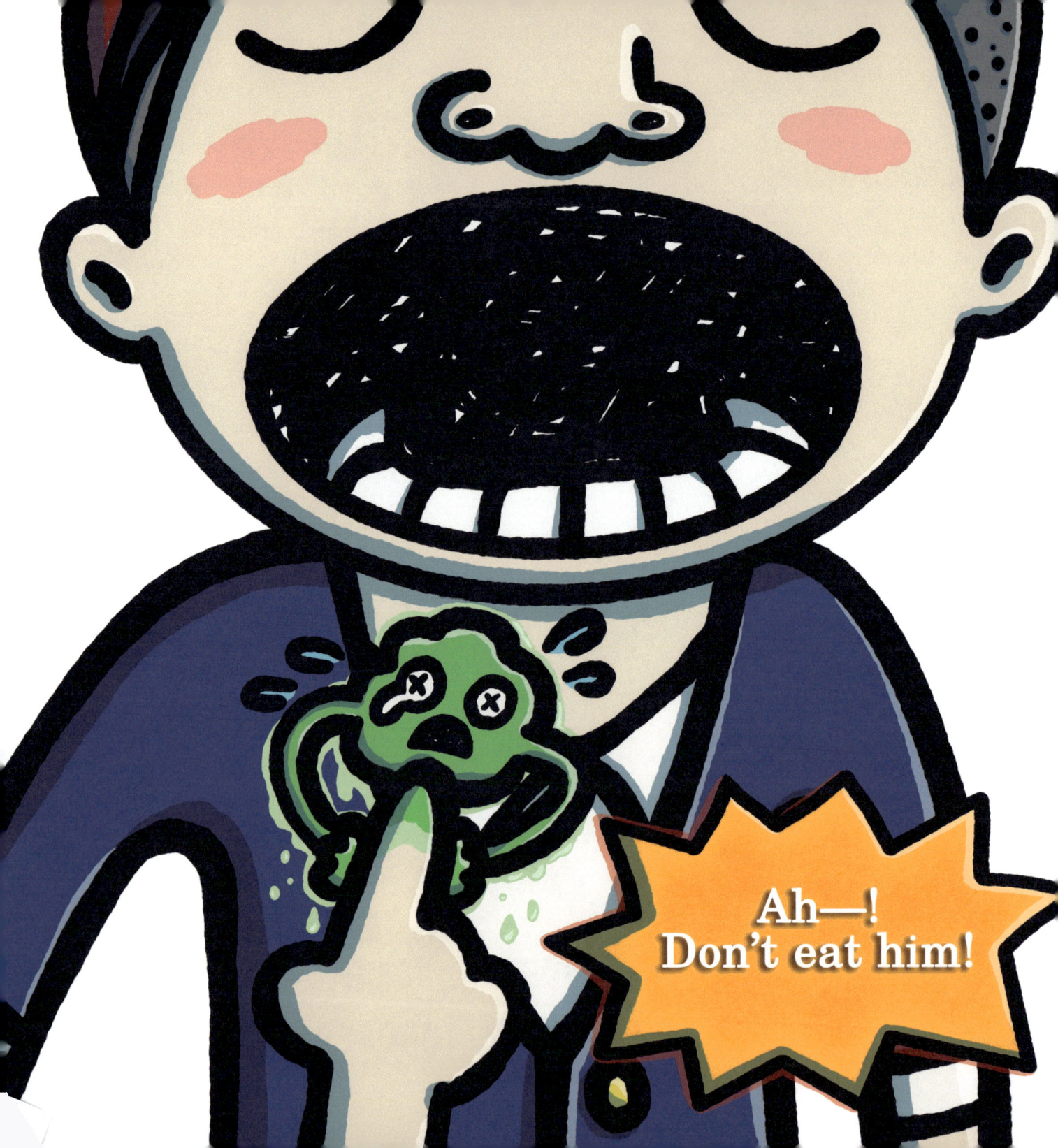

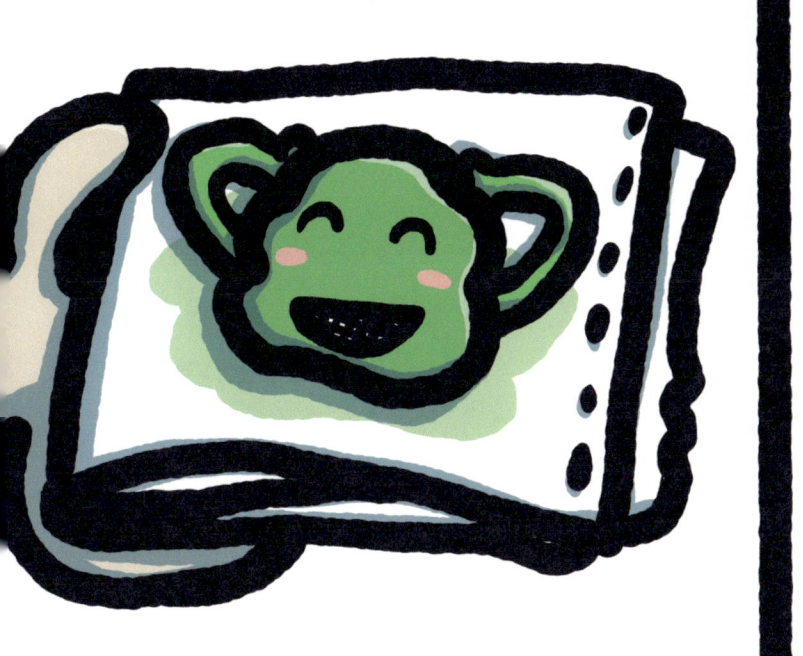

Instead, build him a nice bed.

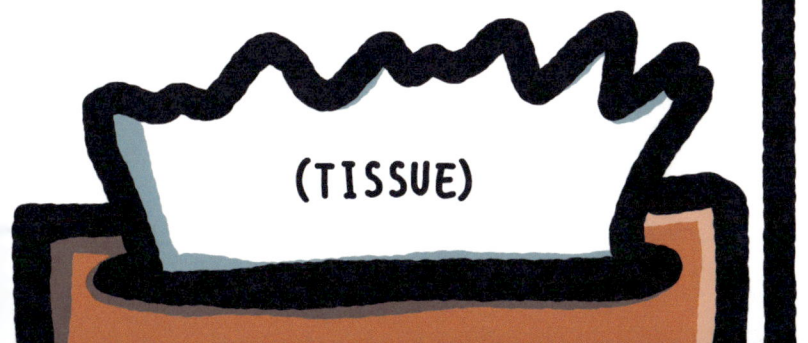

(TISSUE)

And say **"BYE!"**
Bye Bye, Mr. Booger!

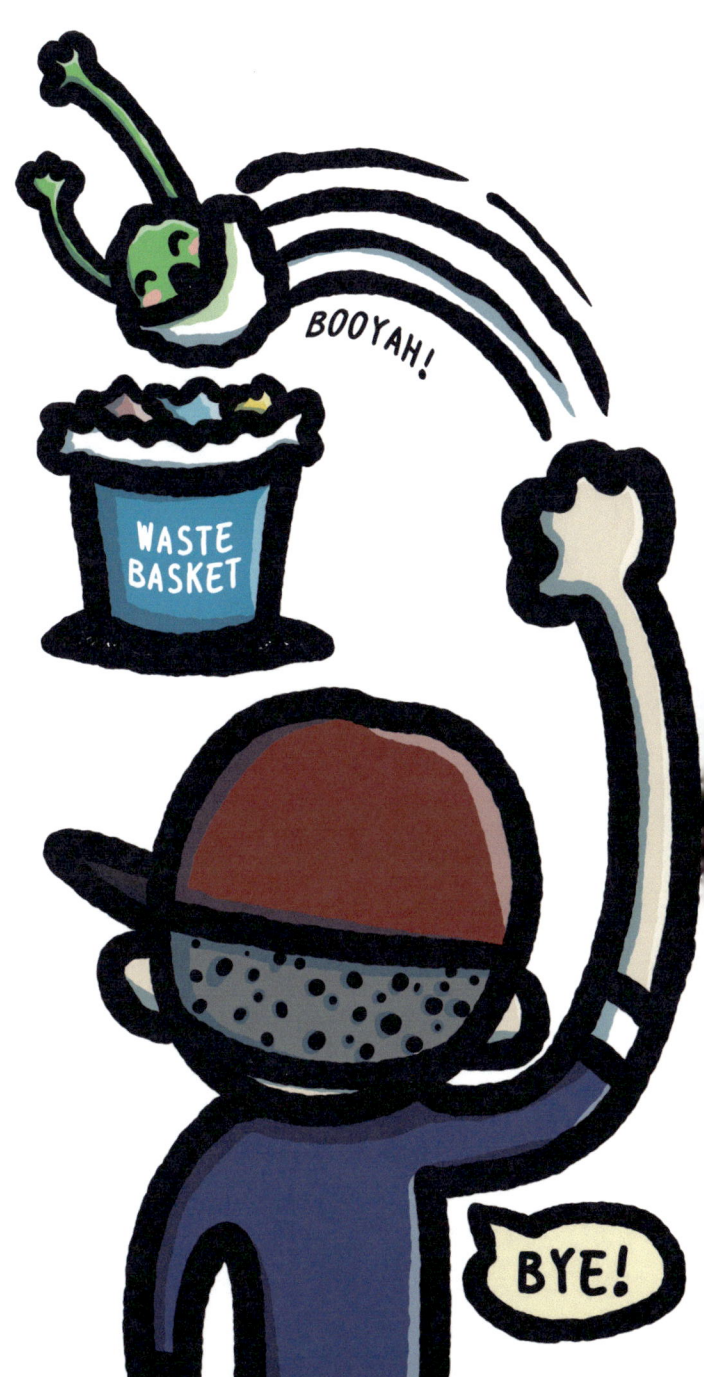

BOOYAH!

WASTE BASKET

BYE!

"Hi!"

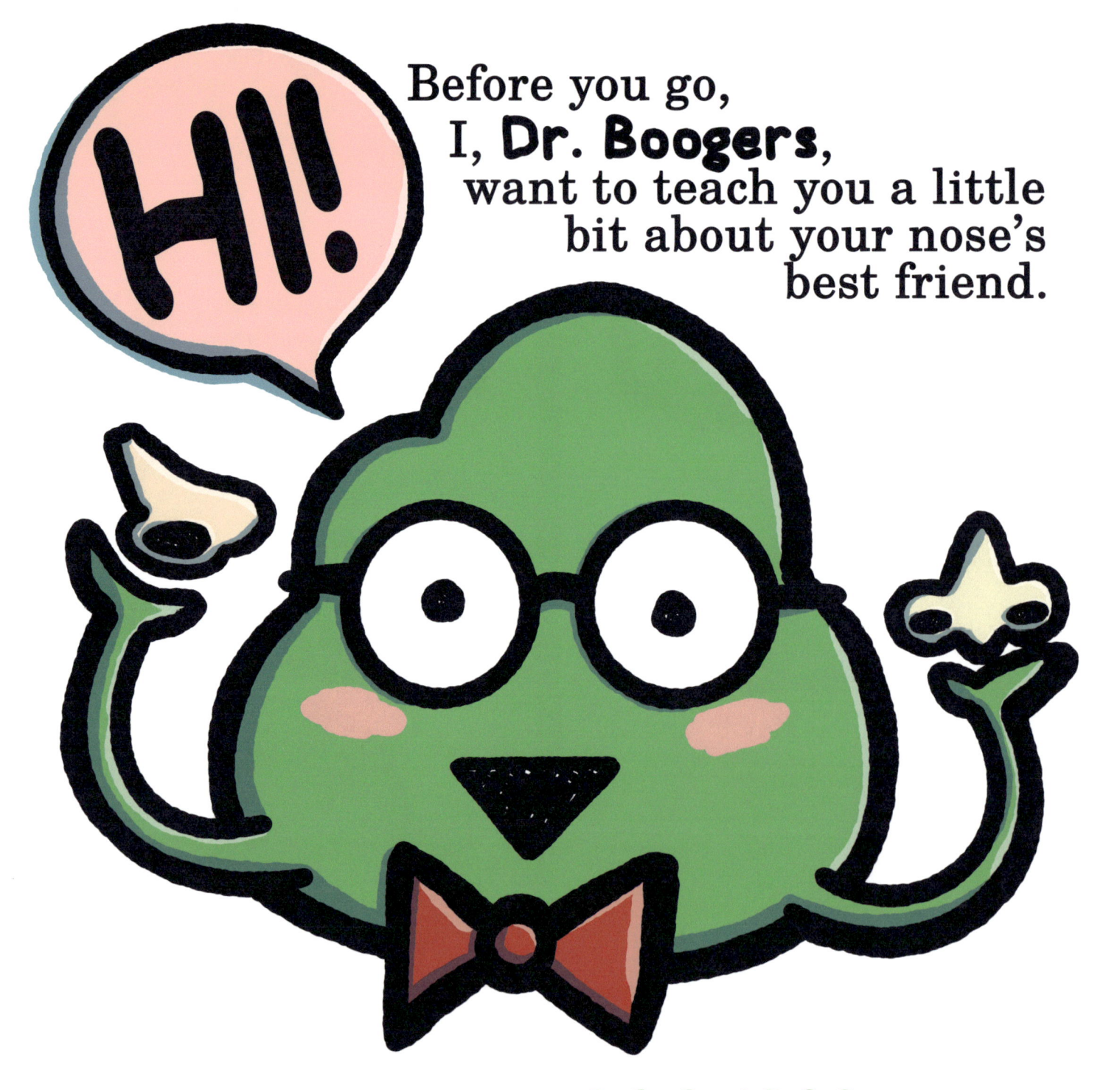

Before you go, I, **Dr. Boogers**, want to teach you a little bit about your nose's best friend.

Yep, I'm talking about **BOOGERS**, of course!

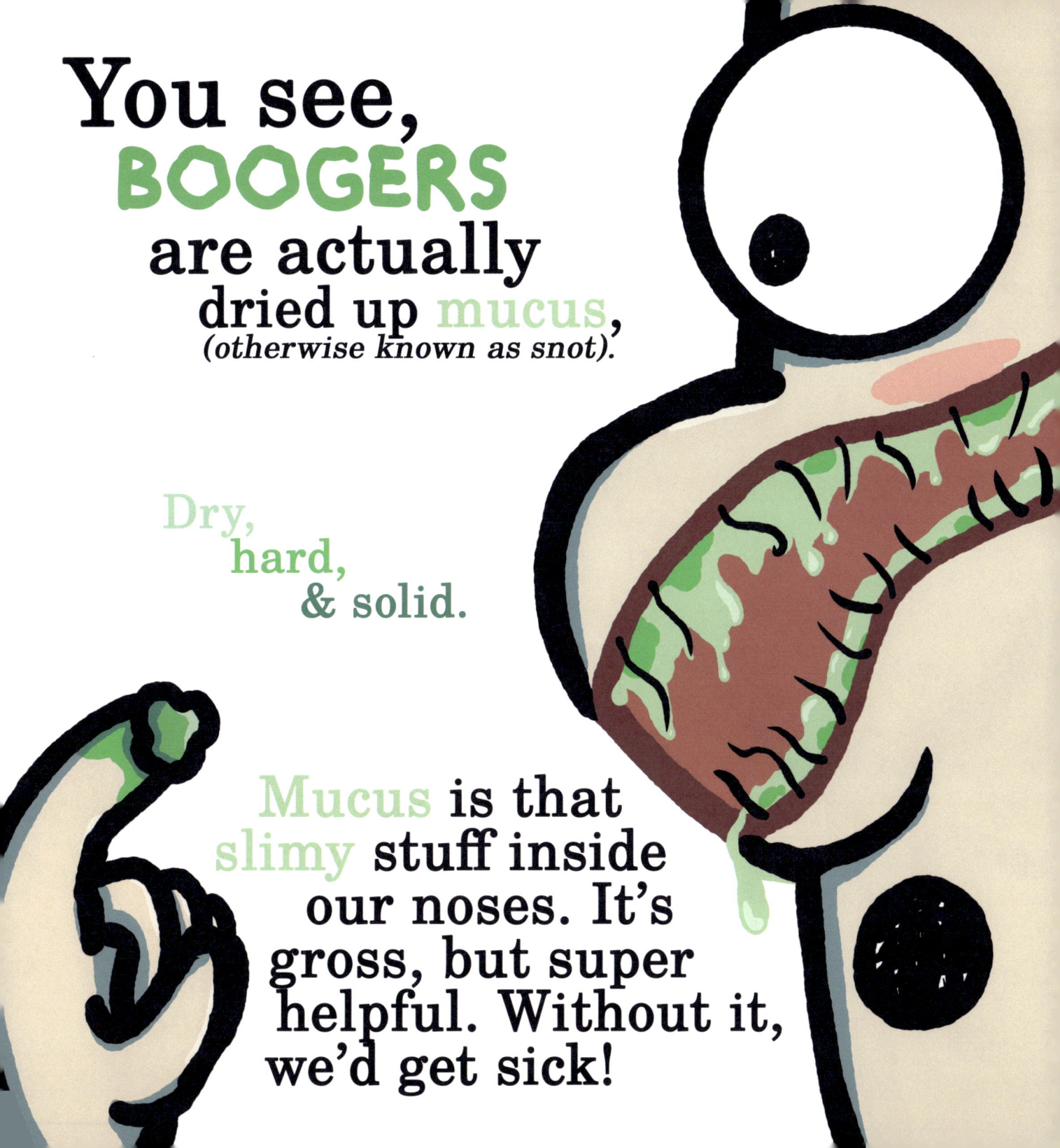

You see, **BOOGERS** are actually dried up mucus, *(otherwise known as snot).*

Dry, hard, & solid.

Mucus is that slimy stuff inside our noses. It's gross, but super helpful. Without it, we'd get sick!

— YOU SHALL NOT PASS!

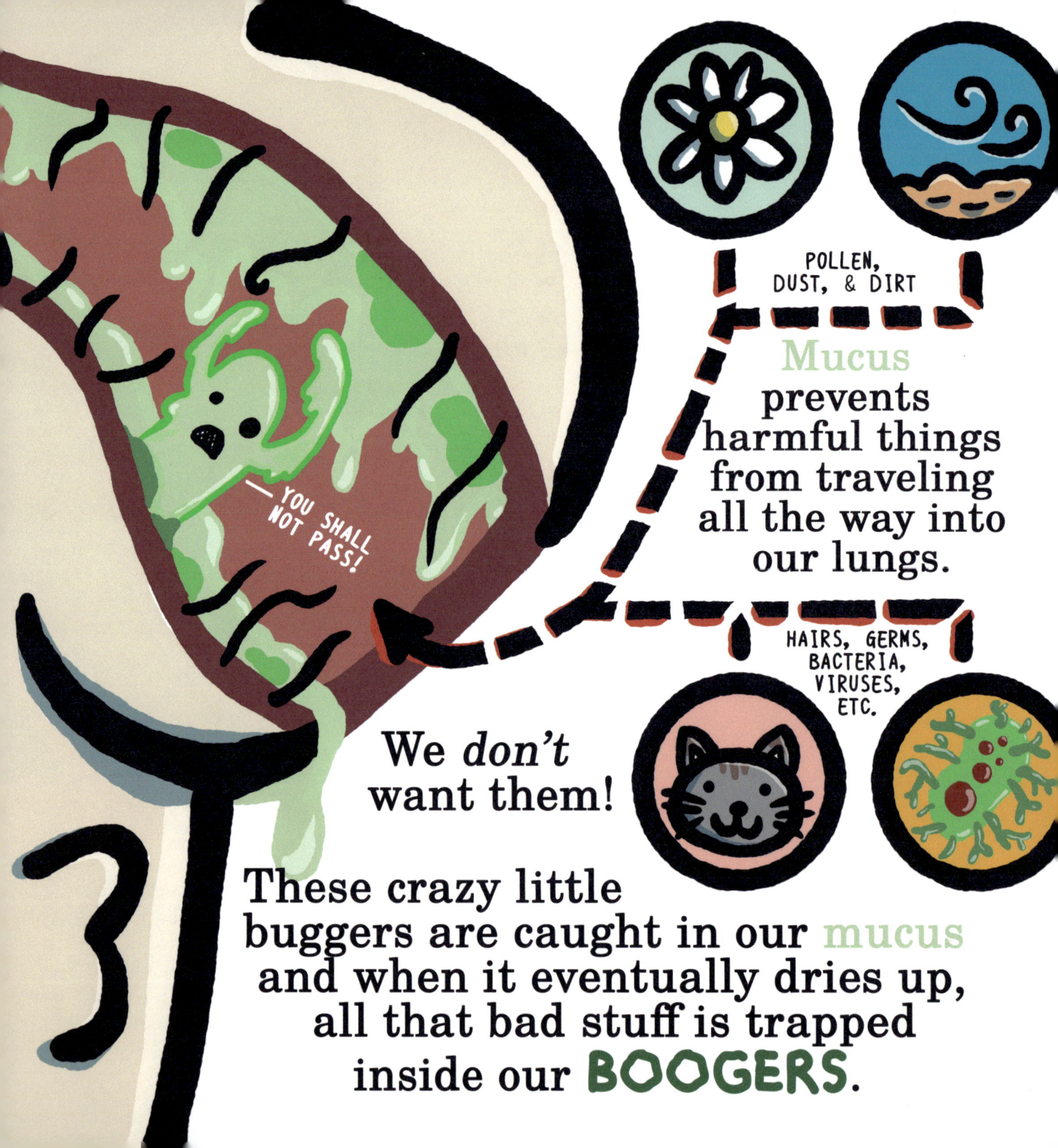

POLLEN, DUST, & DIRT

Mucus prevents harmful things from traveling all the way into our lungs.

HAIRS, GERMS, BACTERIA, VIRUSES, ETC.

We *don't* want them!

These crazy little buggers are caught in our mucus and when it eventually dries up, all that bad stuff is trapped inside our **BOOGERS**.

Some more interesting facts:

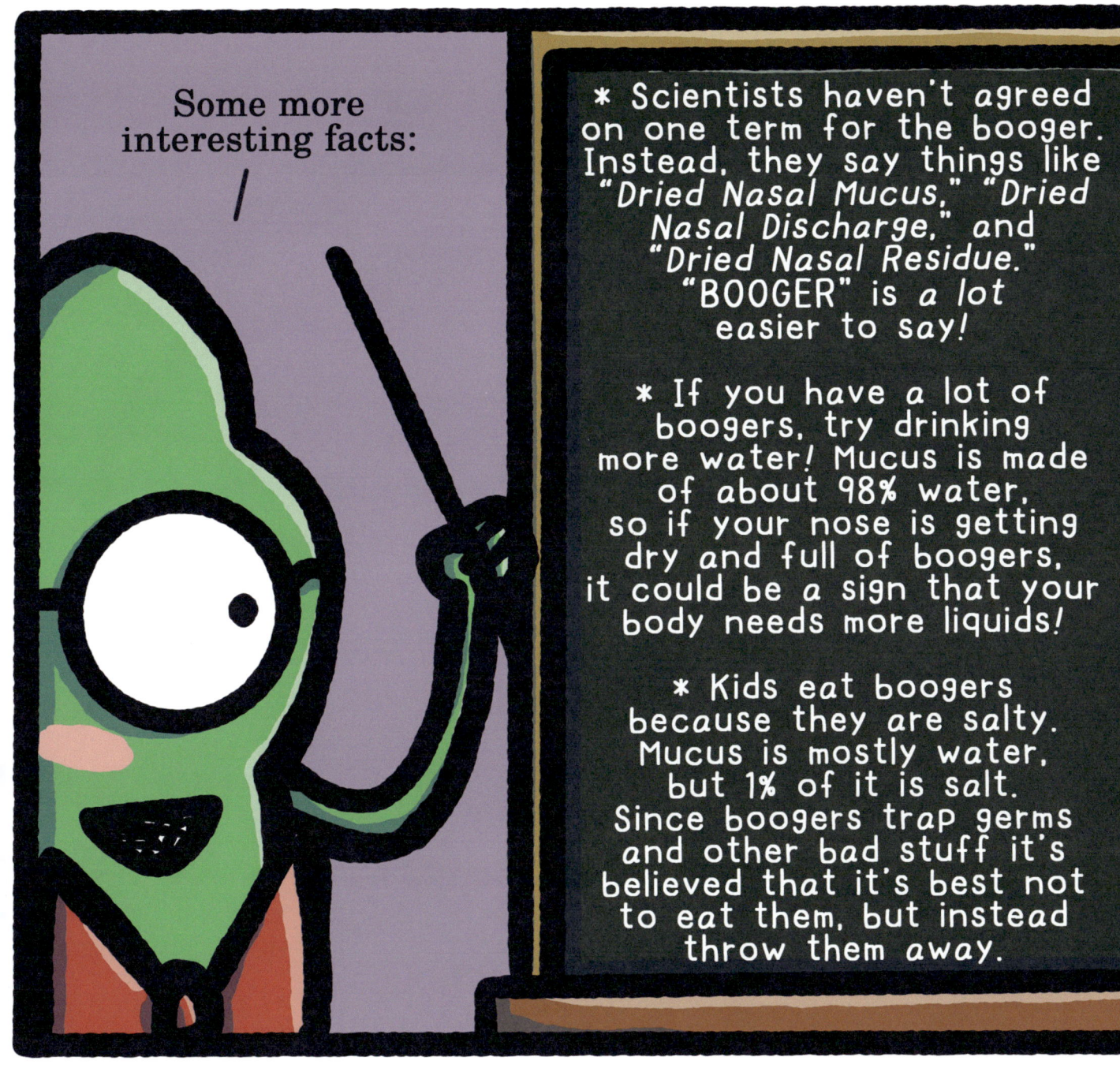

* Scientists haven't agreed on one term for the booger. Instead, they say things like "Dried Nasal Mucus," "Dried Nasal Discharge," and "Dried Nasal Residue." "BOOGER" is a lot easier to say!

* If you have a lot of boogers, try drinking more water! Mucus is made of about 98% water, so if your nose is getting dry and full of boogers, it could be a sign that your body needs more liquids!

* Kids eat boogers because they are salty. Mucus is mostly water, but 1% of it is salt. Since boogers trap germs and other bad stuff it's believed that it's best not to eat them, but instead throw them away.

There's *always* more I could say, but just remember that boogers are our friends—so let's pick them carefully! Thanks for reading all the way till THE END!

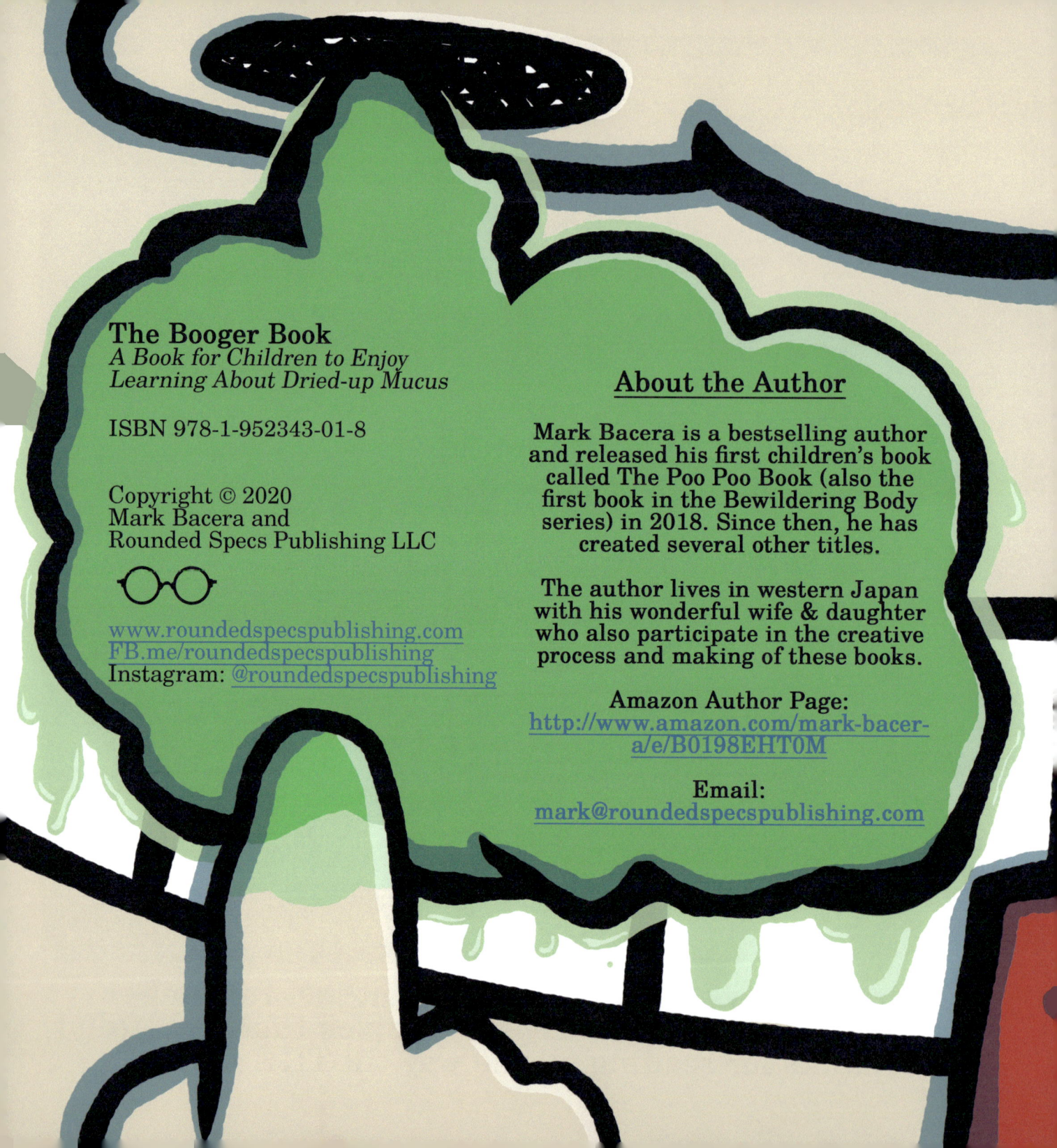

The Booger Book
A Book for Children to Enjoy Learning About Dried-up Mucus

ISBN 978-1-952343-01-8

Copyright © 2020
Mark Bacera and
Rounded Specs Publishing LLC

www.roundedspecspublishing.com
FB.me/roundedspecspublishing
Instagram: @roundedspecspublishing

About the Author

Mark Bacera is a bestselling author and released his first children's book called The Poo Poo Book (also the first book in the Bewildering Body series) in 2018. Since then, he has created several other titles.

The author lives in western Japan with his wonderful wife & daughter who also participate in the creative process and making of these books.

Amazon Author Page:
http://www.amazon.com/mark-bacer-a/e/B0198EHT0M

Email:
mark@roundedspecspublishing.com

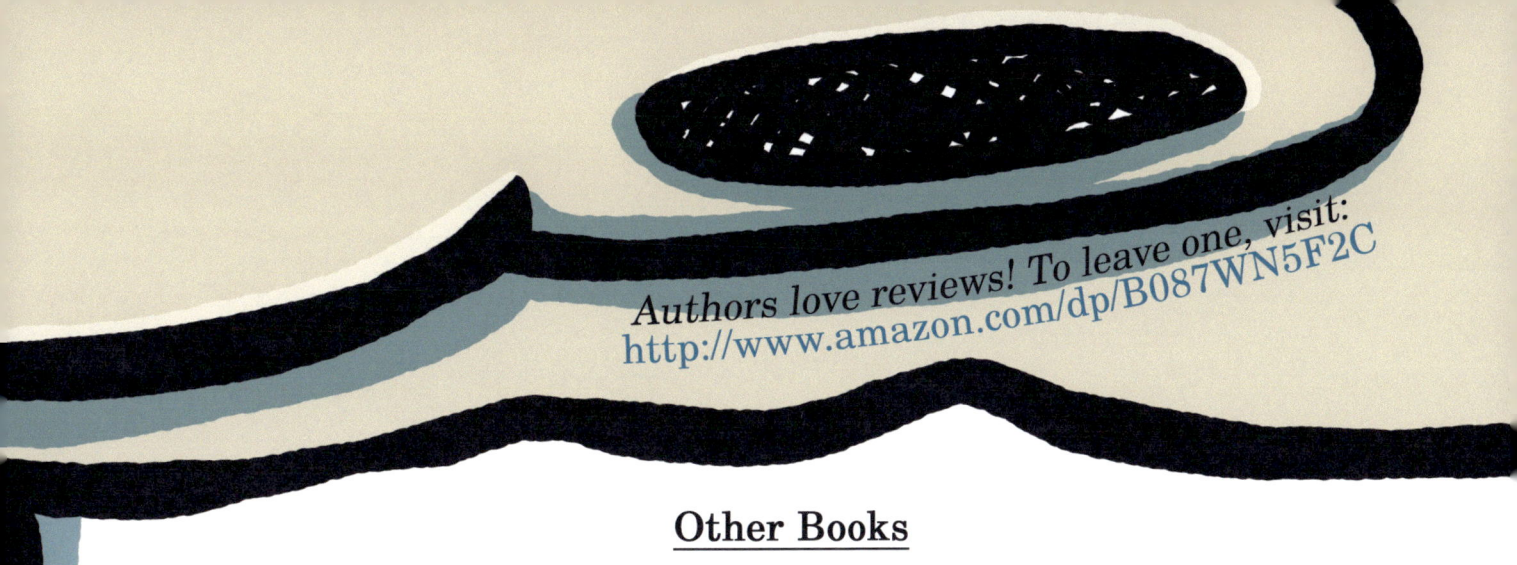

Authors love reviews! To leave one, visit:
http://www.amazon.com/dp/B087WN5F2C

Other Books

By Mark

- The Poo Poo Book
- The Belly Button Book
- The Fart Book
- The Stinky Feet Book
- The Ear Wax Book
- The Sweat Book
- The Tear Book
- The Spit Book
- Baby Poop
- A Naughty Kid's Christmas ABC Story
- I'm an Alien-Vampire and I'm Proud of It!

By Rounded Specs

- A Day With Mae
- Ame the Cat
- Ame Goes to Japan
- Ame Goes to Hawaii
- Ame Goes to the North Pole
- Ame Goes to Egypt
- Ame Goes to the Zoo
- Ame's First Christmas
- Ame's Cafe
- Fashionable Animals
- What in the World Could it Be?

Please note that some of the above titles have yet to be published. To support us and be notified when new books are in the works and released, send us an email at *info@roundedspecspublishing.com*

Made in United States
Troutdale, OR
02/02/2025